Livi **D1076508** Dementia

Patrick McCurry is a journalist and a qualified psychotherapist. His particular interests are in relationship therapy and in the connection between psychology and spirituality.

Overcoming Common Problems Series

Selected titles

A full list of titles is available from Sheldon Press,
36 Causton Street, London SW1P 4ST and on our website at
www.sheldonpress.co.uk

101 Questions to Ask Your Doctor
Dr Tom Smith

Asperger Syndrome in Adults
Dr Ruth Searle

Assertiveness: Step by step
Dr Windy Dryden and Daniel Constantinou

Birth Over 35
Sheila Kitzinger

Breast Cancer: Your treatment choices
Dr Terry Priestman

The Chronic Fatigue Healing Diet
Christine Craggs-Hinton

**Chronic Fatigue Syndrome: What you need
to know about CFS/ME**
Dr Megan A. Arroll

The Chronic Pain Diet Book
Neville Shone

Cider Vinegar
Margaret Hills

Coeliac Disease: What you need to know
Alex Gazzola

**Coping Successfully with Chronic Illness:
Your healing plan**
Neville Shone

Coping Successfully with Hiatus Hernia
Dr Tom Smith

Coping Successfully with Pain
Neville Shone

Coping Successfully with Panic Attacks
Shirley Trickett

Coping Successfully with Prostate Cancer
Dr Tom Smith

Coping Successfully with Shyness
Margaret Oakes, Professor Robert Bor
and Dr Carina Eriksen

Coping Successfully with Ulcerative Colitis
Peter Cartwright

Coping Successfully with Your Irritable Bowel
Rosemary Nicol

Coping with Anaemia
Dr Tom Smith

Coping with Asthma in Adults
Mark Greener

**Coping with Birth Trauma and
Postnatal Depression**
Lucy Jolin

Coping with Blushing
Professor Robert J. Edelmann

Coping with Bowel Cancer
Dr Tom Smith

Coping with Bronchitis and Emphysema
Dr Tom Smith

Coping with Candida
Shirley Trickett

Coping with Chemotherapy
Dr Terry Priestman

**Coping with Coeliac Disease: Strategies
to change your diet and life**
Karen Brody

Coping with Difficult Families
Dr Jane McGregor and Tim McGregor

Coping with Diverticulitis
Peter Cartwright

Coping with Dyspraxia
Jill Eckersley

Coping with Early-onset Dementia
Jill Eckersley

Coping with Epilepsy
Dr Pamela Crawford and Fiona Marshall

Coping with Gout
Christine Craggs-Hinton

Coping with Guilt
Dr Windy Dryden

Coping with Headaches and Migraine
Alison Frith

Coping with Heartburn and Reflux
Dr Tom Smith

Coping with Life after Stroke
Dr Mareeni Raymond

**Coping with Life's Challenges: Moving on
from adversity**
Dr Windy Dryden

Coping with Liver Disease
Mark Greener

Coping with Memory Problems
Dr Sallie Baxendale

Overcoming Common Problems Series

Overcoming Common Problems Series

Overcoming Common Problems

Living with the Challenges of Dementia

A guide for family and friends

PATRICK McCURRY

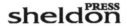

First published in Great Britain in 2015

Sheldon Press
36 Causton Street
London SW1P 4ST
www.sheldonpress.co.uk

The author and publisher have made every effort to ensure that the
external website and email addresses included in this book are correct and
up to date at the time of going to press. The author and publisher are not
responsible for the content, quality or continuing accessibility of the sites.

British Library Cataloguing-in-Publication Data
A catalogue record for this book is available from the British Library

ISBN 978-1-84709-328-8
eBook ISBN 978-1-84709-329-5

Typeset by Fakenham Prepress Solutions, Fakenham, Norfolk NR21 8NN
First printed in Great Britain by Ashford Colour Press
Subsequently digitally reprinted in Great Britain

eBook by Fakenham Prepress Solutions, Fakenham, Norfolk NR21 8NN

Produced on paper from sustainable forests

To my grandfather,
Cecil Lorraine Hawker

Contents

Introduction

This book is an attempt to present an unvarnished picture of the challenges faced by someone who has a loved one with dementia – whether that be a spouse, adult child or other close family member. Much of the support and the literature is about the needs of the person with dementia, but when someone is diagnosed with the condition the close family members are also in need of support and guidance but often don't get it.

What makes me qualified to write about this topic? While I don't have any direct experience of caring for someone with the illness, when I was a child my grandma had early-onset dementia. I would often be puzzled, and sometimes aggrieved, by her behaviour. I'd ask my mum why Grandma had promised to buy me and my brother and sister an ice cream but then forgot and denied she'd ever promised. Looking after her was a long and very demanding experience for my grandad, who was not the most empathic of men. But he had a keenly developed sense of duty and the experience brought out a softer side to him that had not been very visible before.

I have a background in journalism and, more recently, as a psychotherapist. So, having interviewed people who find themselves looking after loved ones with dementia, I have brought my reporting experience and psychological knowledge to give an overview of the emotional challenges faced by people in this position.

The quotes in the book from carers are accurate but I have changed the names of interviewees to protect their privacy.

This is not a book *about* dementia itself, the different kinds of dementia or the framework of support services available in the health service and social care. It is more about the emotional challenges faced by those who look after or who are very close to the person with dementia.

Dementia's ripple effect

Dementia is never just about the person with the illness: like a rock thrown into a pond, the effects ripple out and disturb the close family members of the individual. Those who are often most affected are the husband or wife of the person with dementia or the adult children, especially daughters. Having said that, there may be others directly affected in either practical or emotional ways such as nieces and nephews, siblings and close friends.

Although the book is primarily aimed at relatives who take on a caring role, it is also likely to be relevant to other family members and friends who have a close relationship with someone who has dementia.

This book is an attempt to help carers and family members make sense of their experience and their emotions. Although every person is different and will not feel the same way in response to similar events, I have tried to draw together some common responses to the challenges of looking after or being close to someone with dementia.

I have also tried to give an honest account of how difficult, painful and anger-provoking looking after a loved one with dementia can be. The image many people have of the person with dementia gradually and calmly forgetting things and needing support does not tally with the reality for many people. People with dementia can be difficult, irritating, angry, paranoid and even violent. Understandably, when loved ones show this kind of challenging behaviour it can be very distressing for others around them.

Exploration of emotions

The first part of the book is an exploration of the range of emotions that being close to someone with dementia can generate. Many of these are so-called negative emotions – such as anger, sadness and helplessness. Part of my purpose in exploring these difficult emotions is to normalize them: in other words, to show that they are normal feelings to have in this situation.

If you are in a carer role feelings of guilt can arise if you find yourself experiencing what you regard as 'uncaring' emotions towards the loved one – such as anger.

I believe it is very important to normalize such emotions because much of the message we get from our culture is to hide them, to medicate them or to judge ourselves harshly for having them. The more we can make a place for these emotions in our lives, the less toxic they become.

I have included some suggestions about how to handle some of the difficult emotions and I also include some references to other books that may be useful on specific topics. But this book is not primarily a 'how to' book. Rather, it is about posing questions, exploring what may be happening for us at an unconscious level, inviting ourselves to reflect on our experience.

Relational and psychological aspects

The second half of the book delves deeper and explores further the emotional and relational aspects of dementia caring. Part of this is seeing dementia not just as a medical disease but also as something that has important psychological and emotional meaning, both for the person with dementia and for the carer. That is why I encourage the carer, for example, to view their loved one's unusual behaviour as not simply random acts caused by the deterioration of the brain, but perhaps as communicating a deeper meaning relating to that person's life or experience.

Understanding the history and early life of the person with dementia can shed light on behaviour in the latter years. Unresolved issues from childhood may be reactivated, and carers may be drawn into this and have their own, earlier, unresolved issues touched.

The way in which the person with dementia copes with the continuing loss and deterioration of the illness may in part be influenced by much earlier experiences. This adult–child dynamic can be seen in the relationship between carer and cared-for. The latter is often experienced as childlike, with the carer becoming the adult or parent – a poignant and often painful experience if the carer is the cared-for's adult child.

I also look at how most of us can slip into certain roles in our lives and how these roles can sometimes begin to define us and to limit us. One of these roles is of the 'carer' or 'caregiver'. I look at how this role, while it has a clear positive side to it, can also have a cost. When you become a carer you are no longer that person's lover, spouse, child.

The second part of the book also contains some ways of looking at the experience in psychological terms – I use the drama triangle model to shed light on what can go wrong in the relationship between you and the person with dementia. I also use the theory of sub-personalities to explore how we can reject parts of ourselves, such as our vulnerability or our anger, and then project those parts onto others, such as the person with dementia.

As well as portraying the emotional difficulties of looking after someone with dementia, the book also touches on the potential positives in the experience and how we can develop an attitude of empathy to help ourselves not take personally the challenging behaviour we may encounter.

By becoming empathic, trying to see the world through the eyes of the person with dementia, we can begin to understand some of the unusual behaviour. And in letting go a little of our expectations of a 'normal' relationship we may become open to something new, something different. This could be a moment here and there of calmness and connection with the loved one, an awareness that we can temporarily let go of our everyday worship of time, or a discovery within ourselves of unknown reserves of patience or love.

Letting go of our usual expectations of relationship opens the door so that, in this very difficult experience, there is the potential to find meaning. It is often through suffering that we learn, that we find meaning, even if that meaning does not become visible until long after the event.

Part 1
EMOTIONS

1

The role of emotions

The advantage of the emotions is that they lead us astray.

(Oscar Wilde)

I like this quote from Oscar Wilde because it suggests that one of the important roles of the emotions is to take us out of our rational, logical minds and expose us to something very different, something that is important and often unconscious or only partly conscious.

Writing about emotions and feelings is difficult because there is something mysterious about one's emotional life. In some ways, we are our emotions, or at least that's how it can sometimes feel in the moment.

Although there can be slightly different definitions of feelings and emotions, for simplicity I am using these words interchangeably to refer to the mental state that arises spontaneously, is subjectively experienced and is often felt in the body. It is an instinctive or intuitive experience, as distinct from reasoning or knowledge.

We may ask ourselves sometimes, 'Why am I feeling sad/angry/afraid?' The reason may not be evident, but we know that we are feeling something important even if we can't explain it.

Emotions are also subjective – nobody else can feel my anger, or my sadness or my shame. This can make the whole field of emotions difficult to analyse.

The Merriam-Webster Dictionary defines emotion as a 'conscious mental reaction (as anger or fear) subjectively experienced as strong feeling usually directed toward a specific object and typically accompanied by physiological and behavioural changes in the body'.

Emotions play an important role in our lives. They:

- give us information about what is happening in our lives and our environments, enabling us to make good decisions;
- help us connect with others in a meaningful way;
- can show us whether our needs are being met or not.

3

In neuroscience there is a distinction between emotions and feelings. Emotions are seen as evolutionary adaptations that are non-conscious and in our bodies, while feelings are our conscious awareness of emotions. The amygdala is an almond-shaped structure that is found deep within the temporal lobes of the brain. Brain imaging technology has shown how important the amygdala is in our emotional lives. It is the amygdala, for example, which assesses whether a person or situation is a threat to us and which activates the fight or flight response.

Emotions are often portrayed in a negative way in our society. It can be seen as weak or undignified to become 'emotional'. We may tell ourselves that we should be more rational, that we must not let our feelings take over, that we need to 'grow up' more and behave like an adult.

You will probably find that the medical profession is very focused on the physical and, to some degree, the mental but very rarely the emotional aspects of the person with dementia. When doctors or experts do talk about the person's emotions it is often in referring to them as symptoms of the disease – such as anxiety, aggression, depression and so on.

But people with dementia continue to experience an emotional life, even if they cannot always articulate what they are feeling, and it is important for those caring for, or close to, them to be aware of and interested in these emotions. Because there is often a reduction in inhibition among people with dementia, they can appear rude or aggressive when they are simply stating what they want or need in a very direct way.

So, what are the basic emotions? The experts disagree and there are various lists of basic or primary emotions. Linked to the primary emotions are many other, secondary or tertiary, emotions. Here is a list of some of the main emotions and some of the secondary emotions that are linked to them.

- *Love* – affection, lust, longing, passion
- *Joy* – cheerfulness, contentment, pride, optimism, relief, hope, enthusiasm, excitement
- *Anger* – irritation, exasperation, frustration, contempt, envy, jealousy, resentment, hatred
- *Sadness* – suffering, disappointment, despair, depression, hurt

- *Fear* – anxiety, shock, tenseness, worry, panic
- *Shame* – guilt, remorse, regret.

There is a common misunderstanding that we only feel one emotion at a time and this belief can make it harder for us to describe what we are feeling. For instance, we may tell ourselves we are feeling angry, but then we notice we are also feeling a little afraid or sad, so then we begin to question ourselves about whether we really are feeling angry.

But it is common to have more than one emotion at the same time, although one may be dominant. We may feel very much in touch with anger, but underneath that may be one or more other feelings, such as sadness or fear. So we may have a dominant feeling and one or more sub-feelings, which are there but don't feel quite as strong. We may also have conflicting feelings at the same time – a part of us may feel angry while another part feels guilty.

This happens quite frequently with anger and sadness, and most of us are more comfortable with one of these emotions and less comfortable with the other. What this means is that some people habitually find themselves feeling irritated or angry, but underneath this there may also be a sadness or vulnerability. Others will show the opposite behaviour, frequently displaying sadness or vulnerability but not showing the anger that may be underneath.

Tips for understanding your emotions

- Your emotions don't have to feel large or intense. Sometimes you may only feel a mild sadness, irritation, anxiety. It may feel mild but it is still a feeling; sometimes, if we are not used to understanding or naming our feelings, they may initially feel mild until we get to know them better.
- A good way of handling the fact that we can feel more than one emotion at the same time is using the language of 'parts' of ourselves. So, instead of saying, 'I feel afraid,' or 'I feel sad,' we might say, 'A part of me feels afraid,' or 'A part of me feels sad.' When we say, 'A part of me feels . . .' we are communicating that we may also have other feelings at the same time. In using this phrase we are also saying that we are not completely taken over by our sadness or anger or fear.

- Say 'and' rather than 'but', because when we say 'but' we are cancelling out what we have said before. So we could say, 'I feel angry and sad' rather than 'I feel angry but sad'.

There is a close connection between our emotions and our bodies, and if we pay attention we can usually associate a physical sensation with a particular emotion. For instance, if we are feeling angry we may notice a tightness in the jaw or a tightness in the chest, or for sadness, a lump in the throat or a heaviness in the chest.

I believe that emotions are essential to who we are and they help us make sense of the world and of our lives. Yes, they can be uncomfortable at times and it sometimes feels as though they have taken over. It is scary when we experience wanting one thing with our heads but our hearts seem to want something completely different.

Of course, we must not let our emotions run our lives, but neither should we think we should (or can) somehow use our rational or analytic parts to control what we feel, smoothly rise above it or turn purely to our rational side to make sense of our experiences.

Dealing with emotions can be very difficult for carers and those close to someone with dementia because the whole thrust of the way we practise medicine in the West is to devalue the emotions and elevate reason and science.

Emotions are not given much importance by many people, particularly those who have been in positions of authority in our lives, such as teachers or supervisors. Think how rare it is for someone to ask you, 'How do you feel about that?' after you have described a difficult situation or event. Instead, we are given the message that we should be responding to what others think is important or the 'right' thing to do, whether they be parents, teachers, bosses, older siblings, etc.

As a result, many of us learn to devalue our emotional lives and to view them as somehow less important than logical or analytical approaches. This is particularly true for boys and men, who get the clear message that 'boys don't cry' and who can find it very difficult as adults to know what they feel.

What we feel can tell us whether or not our needs are being met. Underneath a 'negative' feeling is often an unmet need, while 'positive' feelings suggest that our needs are being met. American mediator Marshall Rosenberg has explored the connection between feelings and needs and how we frequently fail to recognize our needs and to get those needs met.

We all have needs – these include:

- acceptance
- closeness
- emotional safety
- respect
- fun
- spiritual connection
- sexual expression
- touch
- love
- autonomy – to choose one's values, dreams and goals
- creativity.

In many ways men are better at identifying their needs and getting certain of them met in a direct way. The typecasting of women as being the nurturers has meant that often women have been conditioned to set aside their own needs in favour of those of others, such as children or family. In the context of carers this is important because looking after someone else and denying one's own needs has been presented as a worthy goal for women, but it can come at a high cost for those concerned.

Rosenberg says: 'In a world in which we're often judged harshly for identifying and revealing our needs, doing so can be very frightening. Women, in particular, are susceptible to criticism.'

People looking after, or close to, someone with dementia can find themselves focusing almost entirely on the practicalities, which means their feelings may be pushed to one side and not acknowledged. This attitude is reinforced by the British culture of 'stiff upper lip' and by the practical and pragmatic emphasis of the medical profession.

Stiff upper lip

Our culture does not handle emotions well. We like folks to be happy and fine. We learn rituals of acting happy and fine at an early age.

(John Bradshaw, US counsellor, author and broadcaster)

When people ask how we are, we often reply 'fine', when inside we may be sad or angry. Many of us, as children, if we were showing sadness or irritation, were told by our parents, 'Put a smile on your face!'

This suppression of emotions is possibly greater in certain parts of the world, such as northern Europe, including the UK. The attitude is summed up by the 'Keep Calm and Carry On' slogan, which dates from the Second World War and was an encouragement to Britons not to dwell on difficult emotions but to soldier on.

This social discouragement of displaying emotion can mean that many people often do not know what they are feeling. Arguably, this is more so for men than women on average.

In a safe place, people are more likely to share their emotions – this may be a counselling room, a support group or having tea with a trusted friend or relative.

But many of us believe that it is somehow putting a burden on the other person if we are 'too' emotional and that we need to be very careful not to embarrass others, or ourselves, by showing too much feeling.

Projecting feelings

Projecting feelings onto the person with dementia may involve us simply thinking that we know what that person must be feeling, even though he or she may not be able to articulate it. We don't really know what someone is feeling much of the time but we may tell ourselves he must be feeling sad or depressed because that is how we think we would feel in his shoes.

This can cause problems if he claims to be feeling fine and we are saying, 'You must be feeling awful, given everything that's happening to you!' He may then feel not fully listened to or understood.

There is another kind of psychological projection which we all use at times to protect ourselves against unwanted feelings or behaviours. It happens when we deny an unpleasant feeling or behaviour in ourselves and instead see it in – or project it onto – another person.

For example, I might be very careful with money but not like to think of myself as being mean. Instead, I find myself very annoyed with a friend whom I perceive as being tight with money.

We can sometimes be so emotionally close to the person with dementia that we can take on, without realizing it, some of that person's pain.

Projective identification

In psychology we use the term 'projective identification', which can come into play when there are two or more people who are emotionally close to each other, such as parent and child, two lovers, or therapist and client. Like psychological projection, in projective identification one person is unconsciously denying a certain feeling or behaviour. But it is taken a step further than in projection, because the person who is disowning an emotion and projecting it onto the other manages to behave in such a way as to induce this feeling in the other person.

So, I may find myself feeling very sad or angry when in the company of a particular person but I can't quite understand why, because my emotions seem out of proportion to the situation. The nature of dementia and the deterioration of the brain mean it is very complicated to explore what might be happening at an unconscious level for the person with dementia, but it can be useful to be aware of the possibility that some form of projective identification may be occurring.

It can work the other way too, so that you as the well person may have certain unmanageable emotions that you suppress and unconsciously project onto the person with dementia. This is more likely to happen if the other person has a propensity to that particular emotion, so for example he or she may be regarded as prone to anger or grumpiness, or to sadness and depression.

If you, as the carer or person closely involved, feel it is not acceptable to feel certain emotions, then it is quite possible some of those feelings will be projected onto the person with dementia. So if you feel you are not allowed to be angry, you may find that the person with dementia somehow absorbs the anger you deny within yourself and expresses it.

Feelings journal

Because many of us are not used to thinking about what we are feeling, or even knowing what we are feeling, it can be helpful to keep a feelings journal. This is just a regular journal that you briefly write in several times a day, if possible. You just write what you are aware of feeling at that moment – it could be some irritation that the person with dementia keeps repeating the same question, it could be a mild sadness about something that has reminded you of how your loved one used to be, or perhaps some anxiety about a forthcoming event.

It is just a place where you can check in with yourself during the day, taking your emotional temperature. You can include how the emotion you are feeling is making itself felt in your body – for example, your chest might feel tight as you get in touch with your irritation, or your breathing might become shallow as you become aware of anxiety.

2

Denial

Denial is a much under-rated survival mechanism. We can face our pain only in proportion to our hope.

(Carol S. Pearson)

People looking after, or closely involved with, individuals with dementia are likely to downplay the reality of their situation at times. This way of coping with overwhelming information is known as denial. It is a natural and understandable reaction and one that we are usually not fully aware of because it is happening largely unconsciously.

All of us use denial in our lives, to help cope with painful situations. By not acknowledging to ourselves how painful or frightening certain situations are, we give ourselves time to digest the information and avoid a feeling of being completely overwhelmed by it. By denying the reality of a very difficult situation we can still feel in control of our lives.

But the problem is that if we continue 'in denial' for too long, we open the door to the difficult situation becoming even worse.

In the case of dementia, it is not uncommon for the spouse or adult children of the person with dementia to close their eyes to the symptoms in the early days. They may tell themselves that their loved one has just become a bit forgetful, that it's just one of those things you have to deal with when you get old, that he or she is just feeling a bit down in the dumps.

Denial as a way of avoiding difficult feelings

There may be a niggling part of us that suspects there is something more serious going on with the loved one's behaviour, but the other part of us insists that everything is fine. The reason for this is that to acknowledge the possibility, or even probability, of dementia is to invite in a whole host of very painful feelings – grief, despair, anger, helplessness.

Susan

When my husband began to show the signs of dementia my initial reaction was denial. I told myself it wasn't too serious, that we had the tools to handle it, we'd been given some pills and it would be OK. I didn't want to acknowledge how this thing would completely take over both our lives.

Former TV presenter Fiona Phillips writes of how she and her partner stopped staying at her parents' home but instead stayed in a hotel when they visited, because the sheets were not being changed or were replaced with sheets full of holes and there was never much food in the house. Phillips interpreted these signs as indicators of her parents not getting on. But they were actually early signs of the dementia that would dominate both parents' lives in the following years.

The fact that Phillips chose to interpret these signs as just a marital tiff was probably in large part because the possibility of one or both parents having dementia would turn her world upside down, living as she did in London while they were in Wales. Understandably, we tend to avoid facing very challenging news if we can find other explanations.

The symptoms of dementia can also come and go in the early stages, which can make it easier to downplay their significance.

There is also the fact that, in certain situations, people with dementia can be very good at hiding their symptoms. In a sense they themselves are also in denial. To a degree, they are able to show the behaviour that they want other people to see, especially those who don't live with them.

So, when the health visitor or the social worker visits, the person with dementia can suddenly seem to engage in conversion in a much more coherent way than usual.

Having said that, it is often only when outside observers see what is going on that the denial falls away. And this can be particularly necessary when, as the caring partner, adult child or other relative, we have become too close to the situation to see the damage it is doing to us.

Disconnection from our feelings

Carers can become so used to the stresses of their role, so used to coping with whatever is thrown at them, that they become disconnected from their deeper feelings and just learn to 'get on with it' because there seems to be no alternative. But the danger of this is that when things are genuinely becoming too much and the carer's own physical and mental health are at serious risk, he or she may not be aware of what is going on.

In other words, when things have got so bad that you are in almost as bad a position as the person with dementia, you need to come out of the denial and take action.

Here are some signs that you may be in denial about the severity of the situation.

- You find yourself losing your temper with the person with dementia more and more often.
- You're not sleeping adequately.
- You're hiding from others how bad things really feel.
- You find yourself weeping or extremely distressed.
- You find yourself drinking more, comfort eating or indulging in other forms of self-soothing to cope with difficult feelings.

At this stage it is important that you talk to someone about what is going on, whether that be a trusted friend or relative, or social services – or both. It is often only when someone from outside sees what is going on that you also begin to see things more clearly.

Martin Slevin, in his book *The Little Girl in the Radiator*, comments on how bad things became when he was looking after his mother and her condition gradually deteriorated. He says that things got so difficult he was in as bad a state as his mother but was unable to see it.

> Early on we'd had some support from social services, but the social worker had long since stopped visiting us and there was no-one else for us to talk to . . . I seemed to spend every day and every night standing with my toes sticking out over a cliff edge. I wonder how much of a final push I would have needed to have gone over for good.

Denial of 'negative' feelings

If we believe that to get through a difficult time we must focus on the positive, we may end up in a kind of denial of what we are actually feeling and experiencing. We may do this in response to messages from our culture around the importance of 'thinking positive', as well as messages we may have got from our parents in childhood that we should smile even if we were feeling sad or angry.

The danger is that if we continually play down or suppress difficult feelings, such as anger or sadness, we can end up superficially 'positive' while actually, deep down, that anger or sadness can become corrosive. If we can't find a way to handle the less comfortable feelings, they can come out in unexpected and sometimes destructive ways.

Denial by the medical profession

You may experience a kind of denial on the part of doctors, nurses and others in the medical profession when they come into contact with the person with dementia. In this form of denial, the medical practitioner is called out to investigate a problem and is minutely interested in every physical symptom but seems strangely to almost ignore the fact that the person has dementia.

Margaret, whose mother has dementia, came up against this time and again in her contact with the local GP surgery. 'My mum would be given verbal instructions at an appointment, which she forgot quickly – something written would have been far more helpful. They've sometimes rung her about GP appointments, which makes no sense because she doesn't know who they are.'

This kind of denial by those in the health service may sometimes be due to ignorance but in some cases it could represent the fear and discomfort that characterizes society's attitude to the disease. Because dementia is not curable and is mostly concentrated in the elderly, perhaps doctors and those they work with unconsciously devalue the person with dementia, frustrated at the challenges involved.

3

Anger

The anger welled inside of me, with nowhere to go. I could feel it eating away at me. I knew if I didn't find a way to release it, it would destroy me.

(Kami Garcia and Margaret Stohl, *Sublimes Créatures*)

Anger is a very basic emotion but it has a bad name in our society. We all feel it from time to time, and if you are caring for or very close to someone with dementia it is an emotion that is likely to make itself felt a lot. This is because looking after someone with dementia can be such a difficult, frustrating and painful experience.

Anger can come in many forms, from irritation, grumpiness and frustration to resentment, annoyance and rage. If you are caring for, or very close to, someone with dementia you are likely to feel angry a lot of the time. This can make you feel guilty because our culture often judges anger as a 'negative' emotion, something that is potentially dangerous or destructive.

Philippa
I feel angry about what's happened to my life since I started having to care for Mum, as well as trying to keep my job going part-time. It feels relentless and it all seems to fall on me. But then I feel guilty about the anger. There's often a low-level frustration, however, as Mum can be stroppy and uncooperative a lot of the time.

But it is important to realize that anger, like any emotion, is not good or bad in itself. Feeling angry does not make us a bad person. This is the difference between emotions and actions. If we feel angry with someone, then we feel angry with him or her. We may choose to express the anger or not. If we feel angry with someone and insult her or hit her, that is very different and not acceptable.

There are problems with habitually holding in anger. Equally, there are risks in expressing it unthinkingly. With anger, there are no easy answers about how to handle it, but becoming more aware

15

of your anger, what stimulates it and how you tend to handle it can be useful.

Repression of anger

Many of us are in the habit of automatically holding in our anger, perhaps because we got the message as children that it was 'bad' to be angry. When this is done over time and habitually, we can become disconnected from our anger and don't even realize that's what we are feeling. And then that anger may suddenly erupt over something apparently trivial. Or it may make itself felt in constant low-level grumpiness, irritation or even illness and depression.

One of the triggers for feeling angry can be the almost constant expectation to be grateful to those professionals or family members who are there 'to help'. We may not be always happy with the 'help' these people supply, but we feel duty bound to show our gratitude. This can create a difficult mix of emotions – we need these people but we can also feel patronized or misunderstood, and there is no clear outlet for our frustration.

There can be damaging health effects when anger takes up residence within us. According to the charity the Mental Health Foundation, there is growing evidence linking anger with a range of physical, mental and social problems. Chronic and intense anger has been linked with heart disease, stroke, cancer and colds or flu. People say that anger is the emotion most likely to have a negative effect on their relationships, according to the Foundation.

The way to prevent anger from leading to physical or mental health problems is, as with all emotions, by finding a means to honour the feeling somehow. By this I mean acknowledging the emotion and finding some means of coming into relationship with it in a way that avoids denial at one extreme and uncontained expression of it at the other.

Research has shown that there is no difference between men and women in terms of the experience of anger, but it is probable that, in general, men are more comfortable showing it than women. This is because society judges women more harshly than men when it comes to displaying anger, so women may find anger a particularly challenging emotion. Women who are caring for a man with dementia, who is likely to be physically stronger, may also be wary of showing anger because of retaliation.

When you are close to someone with dementia you may feel angry when:

- the person with dementia is rude, aggressive or ungrateful towards you;
- you experience health professionals as patronizing, unhelpful or not listening to you;
- you remember the extent to which looking after the person has taken over your life and the sacrifices you have made;
- you perceive family members as unsupportive or uncooperative.

A legitimate emotion

It is all right to feel anger. What we do with that anger is another question, but the emotion itself can play a valuable role in our lives. Anger may signal to us that someone, or something, has intruded upon our boundaries and that we may need to take action. Anger can also provide the essential energy needed to challenge the authorities if we believe someone has been treated badly – either the person with dementia or we ourselves. For example, if our spouse or parent has been unnecessarily left in pain or discomfort while in hospital or respite care, our anger can give us the drive to complain.

Anger at the way society treats older or vulnerable people can provide the fuel needed to campaign for change. When we show our anger we are clearly communicating to others that we are not happy with a particular situation.

The difficulty in expressing anger to someone with dementia

But when it comes to feeling angry with the person with dementia, things get tricky. This is because we are told that her behaviour is not her fault, it is the illness. With a 'normal' person who we feel has treated us badly we may choose to express our annoyance, communicating that we will not accept that kind of treatment in the future.

But expressing our annoyance or anger to a person with dementia is very different because she may not be able to take in what we are saying, or even if she can understand she may have forgotten the incident soon afterwards.

That puts us in a very difficult situation because the person with dementia may have behaved in a way that feels disrespectful or is just downright irritating, and yet expressing our anger is less likely to achieve a change in her behaviour than with a person who does not have dementia.

She may be ungrateful towards us when we are trying our best, or may be rude or insulting. She may look at us with hatred in her eyes or even become physically aggressive.

When these things happen it is highly likely you will feel anger, annoyance or frustration. But because you know it's not her fault, you may feel it's not okay to feel angry. You may even feel guilty about feeling angry. In fact, you may play down your feelings, telling yourself your annoyance is unjustified, perhaps even pretending to yourself that you're not feeling any anger at all.

The danger in this case is that lots of little incidents of annoyance, if ignored, can build up and suddenly come out in an angry outburst.

Anne
I find it so hard not getting annoyed when I have to repeat the same thing again and again or when she's constantly opening or closing doors and windows, complaining she's too hot or too cold. I sometimes lose my temper and shout, 'I've already told you that!' Then I feel very guilty.

The nature of the relationship you had in the past with the person with dementia is also an important influence in how you may experience anger (see Chapter 11 for more about this). For example, if you felt resentful as a child at your controlling mother or father, angry feelings are likely to be triggered when you experience your parent's behaviour as controlling when he or she has dementia. Even though your brain may tell you 'it's not his fault, it's the illness', at a deeper level you may be feeling anger.

Or if, earlier in your relationship, you used to feel annoyed when you sometimes experienced your partner as being clingy or demanding, it is likely that annoyance will surface quickly if you feel he or she is putting unreasonable demands on you, even if you know in your rational mind that it is a result of the dementia.

Anger as a symptom of grief

Having a loved one with dementia is a bit like going through a process of grief because the person you knew seems to be disappearing before your eyes. This is a huge loss and is likely to bring up many difficult feelings. As well as emotions such as sadness, grief can also bring up feelings of anger towards the loved one.

This may sound strange – why on earth would we feel angry with the person who we are losing? Surely grief is about missing that person, wanting him back, so how could we feel anger? Although it seems counter-intuitive, it is the close connection, the love, we have with him that can stimulate anger towards him for 'leaving' us.

But often, if you are feeling this kind of anger towards the person with dementia, it will be unconscious. Without realizing it you may have repressed this feeling. This is because to admit to ourselves we are angry with the person with dementia for leaving us makes us feel like a bad person. We may feel selfish because, after all, he is the one whose familiar life has collapsed, who needs help and support; he didn't ask for this to happen. So to allow ourselves to feel angry with him for leaving us just feels wrong in some way.

But just because an emotion feels 'wrong' doesn't mean we can simply repress it or ignore it without consequences. There are always consequences to repressing emotions. In the case of the repression of anger towards the person with dementia, one possible consequence is that the anger finds another target. This means that you find yourself getting very angry at other people – family members, social workers, health professionals or even God!

Of course, you may have good cause to feel angry with these other people over their behaviour. But if the anger you are directing at them feels disproportionate, that may be a clue that some of it is being displaced away from the person with dementia.

In *Looking into Later Life*, clinical psychologist Heather Wood talks about how some relatives of people with dementia that she has worked with displaced their anger with the loved one onto other people or organizations:

All of the rage and denial found in normal mourning were evident. The ambulance service, which ferried the sufferers to the day unit, was a convenient focus for much anger. Their inconsistent schedules, and the inaccessibility of anyone who seemed to be in charge of the system, engendered frustration and fury in the relatives. They felt as helpless faced with the ambulance service as they did faced with the disease. The former was easier to acknowledge, but making this link enabled one woman to contact her anger that, after years working as a nurse, she should be spending her retirement nursing an ill and difficult husband.

Underneath anger is often sadness

Although many of us, especially women in our culture, are uncomfortable feeling or expressing anger, it can at times feel safer than emotions like vulnerability, sadness, despair or helplessness. For many of us anger is a 'power' emotion, in that we feel powerful when we feel it or express it. Emotions like vulnerability, despair, sadness or helplessness, on the other hand, can leave us feeling small and defenceless.

It is worth reflecting on our anger, therefore, and asking ourselves what other emotions may be underneath the anger. So, for example, the anger we feel towards the brother or sister who isn't pulling his or her weight in caring for Mum may also be covering over a deeper feeling of sadness that we feel left on our own to cope and that someone who we would like to feel is supporting us is not able or willing to offer that support.

Or we may find ourselves feeling angry with the person with dementia for constantly repeating the same question and not remembering our answer. On one level the annoyance we feel is understandable – it can be irritating to have to keep repeating the same answer. But there are also likely to be other feelings underneath the irritation. These may include a deep sense of sadness, or even despair, at how the old relationship with this person has changed. We used to chat to this person, talk to each other about our lives perhaps, but now there has been an almost total loss of conversing with each other – that previous connection has withered.

Anger at feeling controlled

When we are looking after a relative with dementia we can experience anger about feeling controlled by her behaviour. In theory we may be the one 'in control', as we have control of our faculties. She is the one who cannot look after herself, who may be a danger to herself or others if left alone. But being the looked-after person can give her a surprising amount of power.

Her feelings can dominate the emotional temperature of the house; her wants can take over our lives. We cannot do the things we'd like to do because she wants something different and is often not amenable to reasonable discussion.

Persistent demands mean that she can end up getting her own way, as we lose the will to keep saying no.

For example, Mary cares for her husband and he feels resentful that he is not allowed to drive his beloved four-by-four any more because of his illness. If Mary suggests selling it he becomes annoyed and so that vehicle sits, unused, in their driveway while she uses the smaller car she prefers.

> He seems to blame me for the fact that he can't drive any more and is resentful that I still have some freedom. I feel guilty having to tell him he can't drive the four-by-four, or that we can't use the caravan any more. I do my best but he takes his anger out on me and sometimes I can't take it any more, so to stop myself losing my temper with him I get out of the house and drive to a garden centre or country house – somewhere with plants or flowers. After a couple of hours there I begin to calm down and feel better. I'm then able to go home.

Anger at family

Looking after or being close to a relative with dementia can evoke some very strong feelings within the family. For the person who takes on most of the caring responsibility it can be easy to feel that her work is not fully appreciated by other members of the family. The one in the caring role may also feel resentful if she feels that other relatives are not pulling their weight and are letting one person take the strain.

Anger at other family members is especially common where there have been earlier tensions in the family, say between siblings. There is also the common expectation in many families that a daughter will take on the caring responsibility rather than a son. Daughters, especially single daughters, can feel they have had to take on the caring role because brothers, or sisters with their own families, will not do so. This can lead to feelings of resentment and anger at times.

Beware the 'inner bully'

I would argue that all of us are made up of different, and sometimes conflicting, parts (see Chapter 14 for more details). These include a kind and loving part, an impatient part, a passionate part and so on. We are usually more comfortable with certain parts, generally the ones that our families or our culture generally approve of. That means we are probably more comfortable with the part of us that is kind, considerate, upstanding.

We may then repress the bits of ourselves that we do not like, or at least hide these bits from others. These may include the angry part. There may well be a part of us that can get very angry and even tip over into getting satisfaction or even enjoyment from verbally attacking the object of our anger and frustration. Some people may find, when looking after someone with dementia, that they discover a cruel, aggressive side of themselves that they did not know existed before but which is part of them even though it is mostly dormant. This could be called the 'inner bully' or 'inner sadist'.

The best way to handle this part of ourselves is, first, to acknowledge the possibility of its existence. That means acknowledging to ourselves that we may have a part that enjoys getting its own back, or punishing the person who has been making our lives a misery. By bringing this part of ourselves into the open it will have less power.

John Bayley, husband of the novelist Iris Murdoch, describes an explosion of anger that takes on a sadistic flavour, in his book *Iris* (later made into a film). He has been gradually feeling more irritated that Iris continues to water his plants, even though they do not need much water and are slowly being drowned:

> That day I went suddenly berserk. Astonishing how rage produces another person, who repels one, from whom one turns away in incredulous disgust, at the very moment one has become him

and is speaking with his voice. The rage was instant and total, seeming to come out of nowhere. 'I told you not to! I told you not to!' In those moments of savagery neither of us has the slightest idea to what I am referring. But the person who is speaking soon becomes more coherent. Cold too, and deadly. 'You're mad. You're dotty. You don't know anything, remember anything, care about anything.' This accompanied by furious aggressive gestures. Iris trembled violently.

Honouring your anger without being dominated by it

- *Accept the feeling.* Accepting and acknowledging to yourself that you feel angry (or irritated, resentful, frustrated, etc.) is an important first step. You can also remind yourself that the emotion itself is not good or bad and that feeling it does not make you a bad person. Choosing to accept your anger does not mean that it is all right to verbally or physically abuse the target of your anger. It is simply an acceptance that this is what you feel. What you then choose to do with the feeling is another matter.

- *Find coping strategies if your anger is coming out in unhelpful ways.* If you find yourself habitually snapping at the person with dementia or someone else, you may need to find strategies to help you handle those feelings in the moment.

- *Be compassionate with yourself.* I believe it is very important to take a compassionate stance towards yourself when it comes to strong feelings like anger. We are so used to judging ourselves for doing the 'wrong' thing or having the 'wrong' feelings. If you do snap and say something unkind, then, rather than beating yourself up, I think it is far more helpful to be compassionate to yourself, apologize to the person and try and let go of it.

- *Talk to someone you trust.* Getting angry feelings off your chest to someone you trust and who won't judge you can help enormously. This could be a friend, relative or carers' group. Just having the chance to talk about your experience, uncertainties and fears will often make you feel better.

- *Find a safe way of expressing it.* If you feel you need to, there are a number of ways you can express anger in a safe way. These include writing down your feelings, drawing them or even hitting a pillow.

- *Seek further help if anger is erupting in an unsafe way.* If you are worried that your anger is coming out in ways that are physically or emotionally abusive, or that it may do so, you should consider seeking professional support. You could consult your GP about the possibility of counselling or an anger management course or, possibly, some form of anti-depressant.

4

Loneliness and despair

Loneliness and the feeling of being unwanted is the most terrible poverty.

(Mother Teresa)

Loneliness and isolation are huge challenges both for people with dementia and for family members who are close to them, especially their carers. For the relative, the demands of caring mean there is less time and opportunity for seeing friends, for working or for hobbies.

Loneliness is being recognized as a growing challenge for many people in the West. According to the UK Campaign to End Loneliness (<www.campaigntoendloneliness.org>), it is defined as a subjective, unwelcome feeling of lack or loss of companionship. It happens when the quality and quantity of social relationships in our lives do not match our hopes and expectations.

The main types of loneliness include:

- *Emotional loneliness* – this is when we miss the companionship of one particular person who was close to us.
- *Social loneliness* – we feel this when we lack a wider social network or group of friends.

Social isolation and loneliness are not the same things, although they often overlap. Isolation is an objective state in which you have relatively few contacts with others, while loneliness is an internal state or feeling that is dependent on not the quantity but rather the quality of your contact with other people.

Feeling socially connected is extremely important for most people's sense of well-being, not just psychologically but medically. Research carried out at Brigham-Young University in the USA in 2010 found that loneliness and social isolation were more damaging to people's health than smoking and obesity, and were the equivalent of smoking 15 cigarettes a day.

You may face problems such as:

- having to give up, or reduce, paid work, which means less money and less contact with others;
- not being able to go out as much, if at all;
- not being able to go away on holiday or for weekends;
- finding that some friends and acquaintances don't seem as interested in seeing you as before;
- losing the companionship of the person with dementia.

If you are looking after, or very involved in the care of, someone with dementia you will find that your time is squeezed to the max by all the demands. If you are living separately from that person, you will also have to factor in the time spent travelling to and fro.

You may be particularly prone to loneliness if it is your partner who has dementia and he or she was the one who made most effort to socialize, or if you felt much more comfortable socializing as part of a couple than on your own.

Everything is down to you

It can feel very lonely, and anxiety provoking, if you feel that all the responsibility is now yours because the person with dementia is not able to make the same decisions or take the same responsibility as in the past.

Susan

I'm doing all the driving now. We have friends, but many of them live quite a long way away so to visit them means me driving, me deciding what to pack for both of us, including his medication. It feels like a lot of responsibility and has taken a lot of getting used to because in the past all these tasks would have been shared. When I realize that so much of what happens to him is down to me it can make me feel anxious. What if something happened to me? What if I got ill?

Awkwardness with friends or acquaintances

When you do meet friends and others you may find that it is difficult to talk about anything other than how difficult it is looking after someone with dementia. You may find that people you used to feel friendly with seem less keen to see you when you end up talking about the person with dementia.

Andrea Gillies, in *Keeper*, highlights the danger of venting her feelings about looking after her mother-in-law, who has dementia, when she bumps into others:

> I see the tedium crossing people's faces, the light go out of their eyes. I am beginning to repel people. Dementia caring is isolating in more subtle ways than I'd imagined . . . I don't go out of the walled kingdom of the house often on my own, and when I do am very dull company.

One carer, cited in the *World Alzheimer Report 2012* by the charity Alzheimer's Disease International, said:

> As a caregiver it is difficult to maintain outside relationships with friends due to caregiving demands and supervision of the person with dementia. Also your world centres around caring for your spouse and you lose interest in broader issues to discuss with others. Caring for a person with dementia becomes very insular and isolating. You eventually only talk about life in the dementia world because it is so consuming. Friends or family not living in that world may be sympathetic but don't want to hear about the constant challenges of caregiving and the losses associated with progressive dementia.

But the sense that other people are keeping their distance may not just be about the lack of conversation topics you may have: it may also be something to do with the way some other people can react to dementia. I think this is linked to the fear of madness that has been evident down the centuries.

'Mad' people have often been mocked or put in institutions by the state or by their own families, who were ashamed of them. It is almost as if mental illness or cognitive impairment were contagious. Well into the second half of the last century, children who were born with mental impairments were often put into institutions by their parents, with other family members not being told about it. Because the symptoms of dementia in the middle stage often resemble those of severe mental illness, people with dementia can be the targets of society's discomfort with the mentally ill.

There is also the fact that the media often portray people with dementia in the later stages of the illness, which gives the impression that all those with dementia cannot communicate or care for themselves.

According to *Prepared to Care?*, a report from Carers UK into carers' experiences, six out of ten carers found it hard to maintain friendships, although more than a third had made new friends because of their caring role.

Ruth looks after her husband, who has dementia:

> It's very difficult for me to get out because he can't be left on his own for long. Two days a week he goes to the day centre, which helps, but weekends are the worst. I have two children but they live two hours' drive away. What keeps me going is the contact with my cousin, who is nearby, and a close friend in the area.

Despair and depression

Despair is one of the hardest emotions to bear because there may seem to be no hope. It is linked to depression, a feeling of inner emptiness, deadness or flatness. There is also often an experience of life not having any meaning. With depression, unlike sadness, there is often a lot of self-judgement – 'I'm a failure,' 'I'm not good enough.'

Despair often contains elements of grief, anger and helplessness.

Mary
A friend of mine, also a carer, called me to say her husband had forgotten where he'd parked the car and could I help look for it. When we eventually found it she collapsed crying in the street – it was all too much for her. I know how she feels – sometimes I've been out in our car on my own and on my way home thought about driving off and never returning.

Ruth
The worst things are the hallucinations. He sees Germans or Russians in the house and attacks them, knocking over the furniture – he thinks he's protecting his home and me. He also goes through phases of getting out of bed constantly and not getting back in, which means I only get two or three hours of sleep a night. I sometimes feel like I can't go on, and think about driving us both off [the cliffs of] Beachy Head.

I get angry sometimes, especially if he wakes me up in the middle of the night and I'm really tired. I can understand why some couples attack each other. It's like being in a dark tunnel without light at the end and not knowing how long it is. I sometimes feel robbed of my life and of the things I looked forward to in older age.

I don't have any easy answers to dealing with despair and depression. Of course, it is always good to seek support if you need it – talking to someone you trust, ringing a helpline, seeking professional help. But different people deal with these emotions in different ways. Some may use creativity – drawing, writing, making something. Others may find solace in the countryside or in music. Still others will turn to prayer or meditation.

Sometimes it is a matter of enduring the pain. 'I can understand why some people walk away from relationships when one person gets dementia, but my mother told me to stick at things,' says one carer who has experienced despair.

That stoical approach has its place but it is a tough place to be. Perhaps one way of slightly softening the power of despair and depression is recognizing that this is a natural human emotion when we feel overwhelmed, helpless, sad, angry. It often becomes harder to bear when we bring in our own self-judgements and there is also often a feeling of shame attached to despair and depression – 'I shouldn't be feeling this, what's wrong with me?' or 'These feelings are a sign that I'm a failure.'

Despair and depression, while very difficult to bear, are part of the human condition. Sometimes in our culture we can interpret these experiences as a failure of character or of weakness.

But we can choose to see the experience of despair or depression as a call to look at our lives, to look at earlier losses that have not been grieved, sometimes from long ago.

While I'm not wanting to gloss over the deep pain involved, despair and depression can also lead to spiritual and psychological growth and prompt making meaning out of very difficult experiences.

Miriam Greenspan, in *Healing Through the Dark Emotions*, says:

> What our lives teach us is that despair is an emotion that comes and goes, asking painful questions, calling us to go deeper to find a meaning we can live with . . . it invites us to change our lives and ourselves, to transform the way we look at the world. And it moves us to let our grief flow.

5

Intimacy

Losing intimacy, or adapting to a different kind of intimacy, is a big challenge for those close to someone with dementia – especially spouses and partners. But adult children may also find their intimacy with their own partners affected by the demands of looking after someone with dementia.

I am defining intimacy in a broad way, to cover a range of behaviours and ways of relating. These include sexual contact, physical affection and the feeling of shared companionship.

Louise, who cares for her husband, says: 'It's often the little things that feel most important, the things we can't share any more. For example, we don't watch TV serials together any more because Peter loses track. It's mostly wildlife and documentary programmes we have on.'

No matter how old we are, we still need affection, touch and a feeling of closeness. But that can be difficult to achieve when you are living with a partner whose illness means he or she is constantly changing, perhaps including sexual desire or the need for intimacy changing in unexpected ways, and your own sexual feelings will be affected a lot by other changes in the relationship.

The issue of what a husband, wife or partner does with sexual and intimacy needs when the loved one has dementia is a tricky one. There is an understandable sensitivity around this area, which means people may not want to acknowledge intimacy problems to others, even people they are close to.

There is also the message we get from the culture and society that sexuality is generally something for younger people and not really for older people or people who are ill.

Also, a couple's sex life is usually complicated enough in normal circumstances, never mind when one of the partners has an illness that is affecting his or her behaviour in quite dramatic ways.

A couple's sexual or intimate relationship will be directly affected by the rest of the relationship and how they communicate – or not – emotionally. In the early stages of dementia, when the person with dementia is still able to engage in some forms of emotional intimacy, the couple's sex life and/or exchange of physical affection is likely to be less affected. But not infrequently, if the person with dementia is male there can be problems having or maintaining an erection. There are treatments for this, such as Viagra, available by consulting a doctor or other professional.

Some research has also found a high rate of erectile dysfunction among male partners of women with dementia, and it has been suggested that this may be due to the stress that dementia puts on the relationship.

But as the illness progresses it can become harder to maintain a sexual relationship even if the carer would like to. The loss of memory makes it practically difficult because the person with dementia may not be able to remember what he or she is supposed to be doing.

Changing needs and desires

You may find yourself wanting sex, or physical intimacy, but your partner does not. Or it could be the other way round. In both cases there will be strong feelings to handle – such as sadness, annoyance and guilt.

Or your partner may be experiencing so much anxiety and distress that intimacy feels out of the question. The effect of medications may also have an impact on how your partner feels about sex. Patterns of arousal may become less predictable and each partner may feel rejected if the other does not respond to sexual advances.

Some people with dementia lose interest in sex early on, but they may continue to want physical affection such as hugging. Other partners with dementia, however, may experience an increase in their sexual desire.

People with dementia may lose their inhibitions, including sexual inhibitions, and this can cause family members distress. In some cases the person with dementia may behave inappropriately towards strangers in public, use rude language or touch him or herself. If someone is acting inappropriately it is best to try not to react in a shaming way towards him but to try and stay calm and reassuring, while also distracting him or persuading him to move to a less public place.

Theresa

When we're out my husband will talk to anyone and often say something scatological or inappropriate – 'Time to get willies out' or something. It used to really bother me and I felt very embarrassed, but now I just smile and most people seem to understand, although it's harder if it's someone we don't know.

In some, rare, cases the person with dementia can become sexually demanding towards his or her partner. That can lead the partner to feel uncomfortable, and it may be necessary to bring this up with your GP or other health professional. In more usual cases where the person with dementia wants sex and the partner does not, distraction usually works, especially when the caring partner can do this in a calm and non-judgemental way. It is usually only when the partner reacts with anger or disgust that the rejection causes bigger problems with the person who has dementia.

You may even find yourself agreeing to sex as a way of helping your loved one to feel better, even if you do not want it yourself. Again, this can leave you with some difficult feelings afterwards.

Changing roles affect intimacy

But often the caring partner will decide at some stage in the dementia that he or she no longer wishes to have a sexual relationship. Sometimes the reason for this is that you feel your identity has changed. Instead of feeling like a husband, wife or lover, you have now become your partner's carer, or you may feel as though you have become his or her parent. It may be that having to carry out physically intimate tasks for the person with dementia puts the caring partner off having sex with him or her. It is also not uncommon that when the caring partner experiences the loss of an intellectual stimulation with his or her partner and is no longer able to have an interesting conversation, he or she also loses interest in having a sexual relationship.

Looking after someone with dementia is incredibly tiring, both physically and mentally. It is understandable if you find yourself less interested in physical intimacy. You may also feel less attractive when you are tired, confused and stressed. You may feel uncomfortable with the idea of sexual contact with your partner if you do not feel sure that he or she is aware enough to give full consent. Dr Walter Pierre Bouman, writing in the magazine *Geriatric Medicine*, cites research that found 80 per cent of partners reported a change in sexual activity in the relationship, mostly a decrease in activity. In one small study, nearly a quarter of couples in the survey were still sexually active and of those no longer active 40 per cent of spouses said they were dissatisfied with the absence of a sexual relationship. In another study of two groups of couples, in which one of the partners had dementia and the other a control group where neither partner had dementia, it was reported that affection declined in the dementia couples but not in the control couples. Interestingly, affection in the partner recovered significantly when the person with dementia was put into residential care.

The person with dementia may be more emotionally sensitive

But dealing with the partner with dementia's desire for physical intimacy can be a sensitive issue. David Coon, Dolores Gallagher-Thompson and other American researchers into dementia care explore this topic in their book *Innovative Interventions to Reduce Dementia Caregiver Stress* on reducing carers' stress. They highlight that while the person with dementia may have reduced cognitive ability he or she often remains extremely emotionally sensitive and can sense his or her partner's negative feelings. It is important that the caring partner has the right to say no, even if this is accompanied by some feelings of guilt. The caring partner may be able to divert the person with dementia into some other activity or may feel able to respond to the desire for intimacy in a non-sexual way, such as through non-sexual touch, massage or hugging.

According to the authors, there are five areas where caring partners may experience difficulties:

● *Emotional intimacy: having someone to talk to and feel close to.* This can suffer dramatically when the person with dementia's memory is so poor that comments have to be constantly repeated. As the illness progresses, the caring partner feels he has lost the person he could confide in and receive support from.

- *Helpmate: someone to share daily tasks and to discuss major life decisions with.* It can be lonely when you can no longer rely on being able to talk to your partner about big decisions in your life.
- *Mental stimulation: someone you can learn from or raise interesting ideas with.* Many caring partners feel the loss of their partner's intellectual stimulation and all that added to the relationship.
- *Recreational companionship: sharing interests or activities with each other.* It can be hard for a partner when her spouse, who used to be full of energy and enthusiasm for certain activities, now sits in a chair all day. Or for the person who can no longer go travelling or socialize with his partner as he used to.
- *Physical intimacy: hugging, cuddling and sexual intimacy.*

The caring partner will often experience different, contradictory feelings when it comes to the experience of intimacy, or the lack of it, with the person with dementia.

- The caring partner still feels in love.
- In many ways the caring partner has begun feeling more like a parent to the person with dementia than a romantic partner.
- The caring partner feels in a different, new role and is unsure of how to behave. He or she may feel halfway between a spouse and a partner, or between a spouse and a widow or widower.

Feeling these sometimes contradictory emotions may be difficult, but the caring partner may need to find a way through what may seem a confusing experience, in which the caring partner's desire for intimacy may not be fully met, in which the couple will have to adapt to a new reality and in which there may be disappointment and frustration on both sides.

As John Suchet says in his memoir about his wife's dementia, it is incredibly difficult to care for a loved one when you can't even talk about her dementia with her.

Grieving the loss

When you find that you no longer have, or want, a sexual relationship with your partner there is likely to be a feeling of loss. This also applies to the decline of other forms of intimacy in the relationship – the increasing difficulties in sharing activities that you both used to enjoy, the lack of conversation or physical affection.

You are not only experiencing the loss of the sexual or intimate part of your relationship, but also the loss of that part of yourself.

When we experience an important loss in our lives there is a need to grieve that loss. That may mean allowing ourselves to feel the sadness that accompanies the loss. It is by grieving, allowing ourselves to feel the pain that accompanies the loss, that we are able to eventually let go of what we have lost.

Grieving a loss can be helped by talking to others about that loss, but the nature of the loss of sexual or intimate connection means you may feel embarrassed talking about this to friends or in a support group. But it can help to share these feelings with a trusted friend, relative or professional – someone you know who will listen without judging or trying to fix the problem.

Finding other ways of meeting your intimacy needs

When it comes to sexual needs, some caring partners may choose to replace the sexual relationship that they had with their partner with masturbation. This may bring up feelings of guilt, but I would say that unless you have strong moral objections this is a perfectly legitimate way of dealing with sexual feelings. If you can allow the guilt to be there, not get caught up in it and still do what you want to do, the guilt is likely to reduce over time.

Having fulfilling contact with friends or others in your life can have a positive effect on meeting some of your intimacy needs. Being able to connect with other people through a support group or some other activity, such as a choir, church, walking group or other pastime can help meet some of the unmet needs when there is much less, or even no, sex or physical intimacy. Of course, for many caring partners it may be difficult to get out of the house to engage in other activities, and that is one of the most difficult aspects of the role for many partners.

Meeting sex or intimacy needs outside the relationship

Getting your sexual needs met in other ways, such as masturbation, or considering the possibility of a relationship with someone else will often brings up feelings of guilt or being a 'bad person'.

The temptation of beginning an intimate relationship with someone else may occur when you are caring for your partner at home but will probably be stronger when your partner is in residential care.

Peter, in his 70s, whose wife has been in a residential home for several years, has got to know another woman. He says:

> We meet up for a chat now and again and we like each other's company. I think she'd like to take it further but I'm not willing to do that, it just wouldn't feel quite right. My wife stuck by me through some very difficult times in our earlier relationship and so I feel it is my duty to stay faithful to her even though the nature of our relationship has changed dramatically.

One way of looking at this issue is asking yourself what your partner would want for you or what you would want for her, if you were in her shoes. Would she want you to deprive yourself of warmth, love and (possibly) sex because her illness makes it almost impossible for you to receive that from her? Or would she want you to get your needs met in a relationship with someone else?

Of course, it could be the other way round. It could be your partner who begins a new, intimate, relationship in a care home. This situation is tackled in the film *Away from Her*, starring Julie Christie as the wife with dementia who starts a relationship with another man when she agrees to enter a care home.

When her husband, Grant, returns to visit 30 days later, she doesn't remember him and instead has formed a close attachment to another resident, Aubrey. The film explores the confusion and hurt that Grant feels, and the guilt that returns concerning an affair he had many years previously – could his wife, in some half-conscious way, be getting her revenge?

In a twist, Grant ends up in a relationship with Aubrey's wife, who says: 'I thought when I married I'd be with someone till the final stretch – well, it didn't work out [that way].'

The film shows the complicated feelings that Grant goes through, his pain at being forgotten, his jealousy and anger, and his coming to terms with the changes in their relationship. He is also forced to look at the unacknowledged problems and tensions in their long relationship – tensions that are still influencing the present day.

It is not uncommon for a person with dementia to start an intimate relationship with a new partner in residential care, although this behaviour may be difficult to cope with for health and social care staff and family alike.

There is also the issue of some couples wanting to maintain a sexual relationship when the person with dementia enters residential care. A report on intimacy and sexual behaviour in care homes, published by ILC-UK, says:

> When partnerships have formed before entry to a care home, family and friends are often (though not always) supportive and expect the relationship to continue in some way. Nevertheless, some care workers and relatives may be uncomfortable and reluctant to acknowledge or support the sexual aspect of their relationship. The relationship will also have to be monitored carefully to ensure the resident with dementia has the mental capacity to consent to intimacy of a sexual nature.

The report argues that care homes should accept and acknowledge that older people with dementia have a need for intimacy, love and sexual expression. Relationships should be facilitated by allowing regular visits either within the care home or outside, and privacy for residents should be promoted.

6

Fear and helplessness

We are all afraid, deep down, even if we do not admit it to ourselves. We are afraid of illness, pain, loss, not being in control and, at a much deeper level, of death. Feeling fear is part of being human.

But people with dementia, and the family members close to them, can face an additional level of fear. Linked to this fear is a more generalized anxiety and helplessness about, among other things, the relentless progression of the disease. This does not mean that there are not happy, lighter moments, but often in the background lurks the fear of what the future holds.

It can be very difficult for us to allow ourselves to feel fear, anxiety or helplessness, or to show it. This is, in large part, because we live in a culture in which these feelings are deemed 'negative'. They are uncomfortable, sure, but like all emotions they have a role and it is often the interpretation that we put on them that makes them damaging. If we immediately judge our fear, anxiety or helplessness as something bad, as something that shows we are a not-good-enough person or carer, then we turn an uncomfortable feeling into a more powerful and potentially damaging one.

Fear and helplessness can begin early on.

Keith

It took me and my sister a long time to get a diagnosis for Mum, and then when the consultant asked me what questions I had I couldn't think of anything – it all felt so overwhelming and I didn't have a clue what to ask about. What I really wanted was for him to tell me what I should ask. At the beginning I didn't feel supported at all, which was scary and disorientating. It was only after I spoke to people at the Alzheimer's Society that I got more of an idea about what the future held, but with officials in social services it's hard to get a straight answer. The hardest things for me have been the guilt and the helplessness.

Fear is a side effect of the illness

Richard Taylor, an American psychologist, has written about his experiences of early-onset dementia in *Alzheimer's From the Inside Out*. He says:

> The diagnosis has a side effect that is not listed in any of the drug pamphlets. It is fear! We all live with fear: spouses, family members, friends and of course yours truly. Fear has contaminated our hearts, minds, and feelings. It's worse than cancer because we can't cut it out. We can't kill it with radiation. We cry, we get mad, we get sad, and we get scared.

Oliver James, who explains his mother-in-law Penny Garner's approach to helping people with dementia in the book *Contented Dementia*, describes the acute fear that someone with dementia feels when she realizes she is forgetting things. He compares the process of a person with dementia forgetting things to having a photo album in which the photos gradually disappear, while the feelings associated with the events in the photos remain.

In his example, Arthur asks his wife Dolly to post a letter for him. Dolly puts the letter in her handbag but then, because of the dementia, forgets all about the conversation. When Arthur later asks her if she has sent the letter she has no recollection of the conversation and says he never asked her to post anything. Arthur becomes angry about this, while Dolly thinks Arthur must be going mad to bring up non-existent conversations. When Arthur takes the letter out of Dolly's handbag she becomes filled with panic.

James says:

> A serious threat to her emotional well-being has arisen. As she contemplates the new and strange situation an unbearable panic develops on a scale she has never known before. Another person, her husband, has facts about her recent activity in his [photo] album that should also be in hers. She had no idea of this until he pointed it out, but now she is fully aware. Massive ill-being follows as she considers what other information she may, unknowingly, have failed to store. She realises that she may never know how many other times this has happened. Meanwhile, Arthur has no idea of what she is going through.

This experience severely dents her self-confidence and, as more of these kinds of incidents happen, her life is filled with increasing panic and anxiety, which family members around her cannot completely understand.

So, people with dementia experience a great deal of fear – of the future, of the unknown, of losing their minds and of dying. And you also will feel much of this fear even if for much of the time you may not be aware of it because you will be covering it over with busyness, practicalities and day-to-day tasks.

You will also almost certainly go through periods of feeling helpless or trapped – helpless, because there is nothing you can do to cure your loved one of dementia. If you are caring for him or her you may feel trapped in this responsibility, having to sacrifice your own wants and needs in order to take on someone else's care and well-being.

Specific fears

There are specific fears that you may have, such as how your family member will cope in hospital or in respite care. Will he be looked after appropriately? Will her needs be met? What will become of your career, if you have given it up to become a carer? Will your financial situation worsen? Will the person with dementia have hallucinations tonight or get up and refuse to go back to bed?

These are all specific and understandable fears. But there is also a less specific, more generalized fear that you may have and that is present in the culture at large. I think this is a fear of decay and death – a fear that we try to keep out of conscious awareness most of the time, as we distract ourselves with busyness, being productive and consumption. Our culture focuses on the young, on beauty and on health. It is far less comfortable with ageing, illness and death.

When you are looking after, or close to, someone who is visibly deteriorating and on a path to death it is difficult not to sometimes think of your own decline and future death, which is a thought most of us tend to put out of our minds. It is difficult to watch someone decline through a progressive and terminal illness without recognizing, at some level, that you too will die, perhaps even in the same way. If it is a parent who has dementia, the knowledge that he or she is dying can bring home the fact that soon you will be part of the next generation to die.

Mary
My husband's personality has changed and is less predictable and that can lead to stress for me. The hard part is knowing what is coming next – he can sit quietly for three days or suddenly become aggressive. I also feel fear about the future. I attend a carers' group and so hear about some of the other spouses with dementia and what their behaviour is like and that can feel frightening.

Anxiety

Anxiety is a form of fear, worry and uneasiness that tends to be unfocused and generalized. It is more of an underlying feeling that something bad might happen. Symptoms of anxiety include difficulties sleeping, high levels of worrying, tiredness and mental stress. We can feel irritable, jumpy or on edge. Physical symptoms may include heart palpitations, shortness of breath and lightheadedness.

You probably have good cause to experience anxiety because the person with dementia may have behaved unpredictably and you don't know what the next incident will be or where and when it will happen.

You may experience particular anxiety if you've had to handle your loved one behaving in an aggressive or self-destructive way. The knowledge that some form of aggression or frightening behaviour can erupt suddenly can to lead to a more generalized anxiety.

Anxiety can also arise as a result of the extra responsibility we may have, with regard to managing other people's feelings concerning the person with dementia.

Susan
As a carer one of the hardest things is having to deal with other people if my husband has forgotten who they are. I have to try and handle the situation so that they don't feel too bad. Most people now know that they can't talk to him on the phone and expect him to pass on information to me, but it's hard for them to accept this because he puts on such a good front.

People often think he's remembered them but it's because he's so good at pretending and asking them questions about themselves. I find it stressful trying to manage other people's expectations and feelings.

How can we deal with our fear?

Fear, like all emotions, can play a positive role in our lives. It is fear of how our loved one may be treated in residential care that makes us take a lot of time to find the right care home, where we feel confident of good-quality care. It is fear that we may be approaching burn-out that encourages us to explore other options of looking after the person with dementia. These are examples of the necessary and positive role that fear can play.

First of all we need to accept it. Much as fear is an uncomfortable and even unpleasant emotion, the more we can allow it to be present without letting it take over, the better.

If we can make friends with our fear it will have less power over us. The more we put it to the back of our minds, distract ourselves or tell ourselves we're not really afraid, the stronger it will be. If we can allow ourselves to feel it, by breathing into it and becoming aware of where we feel it in our body, we will be able to open ourselves to what it is there to teach us. That teaching may be that we are vulnerable, that we are mortal, that life is impermanent or that we are not in control.

Feeling trapped

The all-enveloping nature of being with, or looking after, someone with dementia can lead to a feeling of being trapped. Chris Carling in *But Then Something Happened* describes how her mother's condition worsened and her behaviour became more worrying and confused. Carling says, looking back, she was operating on two levels – one in which she remained the same matter-of-fact daughter coping with Mum's odd behaviour, and a deeper level of anguish and anxiety that she did not often admit to herself, which she compares to 'being trapped in a brightly lit cellar'.

You can sometimes feel as though the person with dementia has taken over your life, leaving you with very little real independence. A daughter on the Alzheimer's Society internet forum describes how she and her husband and young daughter have moved in with her mother, who has dementia, because they are worried Mum cannot cope on her own. But this arrangement isn't working, with the mother interfering in the relationship between the daughter and her child. 'I feel like Mum is emotionally blackmailing me, but I know she doesn't intend to. I am finding it impossible as a sandwich carer and feel my daughter is missing out on a normal upbringing.'

Helplessness

This is similar to feeling trapped and is one of the most difficult feelings for us, as we are brought up in a culture that tells us we should be in control of our lives, that we should be strong (not weak), independent (not needy). But in the face of a loved one slowly dying from an incurable and progressively disabling illness it is hard not to sometimes feel helpless.

There are many times when you may feel helpless, such as when:

- you have no idea how to handle certain behaviour from the person with dementia;
- you do not live with the person with dementia and must rely on others to provide essential care and support;
- you have to stand by and watch the person gradually deteriorate;
- your advice or support is ignored or not understood by the person with dementia;
- no matter how hard you try, you can't seem to get the right kind of support or care for the person with dementia.

Feeling helpless or powerless is a very difficult emotion to experience. Our instinct is to look for a solution, something that we can 'do' – anything rather than be left with this feeling of helplessness.

Many of us spend a lot of time and energy constructing lives in which we try to banish helplessness and vulnerability. Spending time with a person with dementia puts us in touch with that deeper insecurity and helplessness that is part of being human.

Family carer Keith, who looks after his mother, says: 'One of the hardest feelings is the impotence – watching a loved one deteriorate with dementia is a lonely experience.'

People who are 'doers', who value themselves in terms of what they do and what they achieve, are probably going to find the inevitable experiences of helplessness harder to cope with. This is because, for them, the process of 'doing something', providing a solution, making things better, is a way of not facing the deeper pain and despair of being close to someone whose brain is slowly being destroyed with dementia.

Fear of dependency

As the disease develops, the person with dementia becomes increasingly dependent and helpless. This can activate one's own fears of getting old and infirm and becoming dependent on others. Fear of dependency in old age can be linked to an earlier experience of being dependent and not having one's needs met.

For some of us, our needs were not met as a baby or infant. This may have been because our mother or primary carer was depressed, emotionally unstable or inconsistent in our care. If that was our experience as a child we are likely to have taken in a message that we cannot really rely on other people to care for us. That can leave us feeling extremely uncomfortable and disturbed when we imagine being unable to take care of ourselves and having to be dependent on others.

When we find ourselves looking after, or in close contact with, someone with dementia, our own fears of being dependent on others can be triggered. We may not be fully conscious of these fears or of our own dependency issues, but they may make themselves felt through a more generalized fear or anxiety.

Some ways of handling your helplessness:

- Allow yourself to feel the feeling, without panicking. Helplessness is an uncomfortable emotion, so allow yourself to breathe into it. You can allow it to be present without having to fight it, suppress it or get caught up in it.
- Remind yourself that you are not all-powerful and that sometimes you have to let go of your desire to fix things or take away someone else's pain.
- Remember that there is a time to be active and a time to be still. You will have often been able to take action, to help, support and advise. But part of the process of dementia is recognizing that it is beyond your control and there will be times when acceptance of how things are cannot be avoided.

When I think of helplessness, the serenity prayer comes to mind. This is a prayer written by American theologian Reinhold Niebuhr, which has become very popular in Alcoholics Anonymous and other 12-step recovery groups:

God, grant me the serenity
to accept the things I cannot change,
the courage to change the things I can,
and the wisdom to know the difference.

7

Guilt

Feeling guilty a lot of the time seems to be part and parcel of helping care for a family member with dementia. Many of us, carer or non-carer, are gluttons for self-punishment, and it doesn't take much to get us feeling guilty. But while sometimes guilt can be appropriate, it can often be corrosive to our self-esteem and actually damage the relationship with the person with dementia.

Healthy and inappropriate guilt

I would distinguish between two types of guilt:

- *Healthy guilt.* This is when we have done something that goes against our beliefs and values. We are able to recognize that we have done something wrong, admit it and make amends where possible. Often we feel healthy guilt when we have done something that damages relationships that are important to us or that damages our relationship with our deeper self or our self-esteem.
- *Inappropriate guilt.* This is to do with the commands or beliefs of others which we have somehow taken on within ourselves, often without realizing. We may find ourselves feeling guilty at breaking these judgements that have been imposed by others.

The difference between healthy guilt and inappropriate guilt is that with healthy guilt we can acknowledge that we have made a mistake, make amends or put it right if possible, and move on. Inappropriate guilt, however, focuses on blame and judging. If we are subject to feeling inappropriate guilt we are likely to seek to be perfect and not allow ourselves any room for mistakes or imperfection.

As one carer says: 'My biggest emotional problem is the guilt – I feel I never do enough. However long I visit my mother for, I feel it should be longer.'

It can sometimes feel as though inappropriate guilt is something you carry around with you. It may feel like this because the origins of this kind of guilt often go way back to childhood.

Guilt about not being perfect

Some of us can feel that everything that happens to the person with dementia is somehow our responsibility. We may know rationally that we can't be expected to do everything but, at a deeper emotional level, we feel we should and we can beat ourselves up when we think we've failed in some way.

There are several possible reasons why we may take too much responsibility. One is that, when a child, we didn't feel we got as much love or attention from one or both our parents as we wanted. A child in that situation can take in the message 'There is something wrong with me,' and thus try to be perfect in order to win approval.

Of course, if we think about it we know that nobody can be perfect, but we still aim for this unattainable goal and when we fall short, as we inevitably will, we feel a deep sense of guilt.

Guilt about anger

Inappropriate guilt often covers over something else that we are uncomfortable with. One of the most common examples of this is feeling guilty about certain thoughts or feelings. These may include feeling angry at the person with dementia.

I believe that our thoughts and feelings are never good or bad in themselves. It is what we do with those thoughts and feelings – in other words, our actions – that matters. So, if we are feeling angry with the family member that is just a feeling, neither good nor bad. But if we feel angry and hit that person, that is violence and abuse and we will almost certainly feel healthy guilt.

It is not the feeling angry that is the problem. We feel what we feel. It is what we do with that feeling that matters. We can try to find a way of handling that feeling in a way that is not destructive or abusive, or we can blame the person with dementia and take it out on him or her. We have a choice.

Fernanda
It became clear that someone would have to accompany my mum to any doctor or other appointment and I ended up taking on that role. I felt annoyed about taking on someone else's social, personal and financial affairs, especially because my mum made it clear she felt she didn't need any help. This all led to a feeling of guilt on my part about these feelings.

Guilt is sometimes described as anger turned inwards. We may feel we don't have the right to feel angry with this person, who may have taken over our lives, because he or she is our parent or partner and can't help this behaviour. But when those legitimate feelings of anger are shut down because we judge them as bad, that anger can be turned on ourselves and take the form of inappropriate guilt.

As David Richo says in *How to Be an Adult,*

> Guilt can mean justifiable anger toward a respected parent, authority figure or friend who seems to have obligated or inhibited us. We believe it is unsafe or wrong to feel or to express this anger. This leaves only us to be wrong and so the unexpressed anger turns inward as guilt.

Many of us have been brought up in families where we were told it was 'wrong' to feel anger. This is especially true for girls. So when we feel angry, that triggers a feeling of guilt. But the problem is not feeling angry, which is a normal and legitimate emotion, but the belief or judgement that we have internalized that we are somehow 'bad' for feeling it.

We may tell ourselves that the person with dementia cannot help himself, that it is the disease that is making him behave in such a difficult way. Then when we feel irritated or annoyed we may feel guilty because we know it's not his fault. But we are human and we don't like being taken for granted or feeling ignored or controlled. Some form of anger is an understandable feeling to have in response to this kind of behaviour.

We may find ourselves losing our control sometimes and saying things we regret, and this is an opportunity for healthy guilt, for saying sorry and moving on. It is better to find a way of honouring this legitimate anger without habitually losing your temper with the family member (see Chapter 3 on anger).

Guilt at feeling relief or enjoyment

When the person with dementia is away, in respite care or having moved into a care home, there is likely to be a part of us that feels relief or happiness about this. But there may also be another part of us that judges we should not have these kinds of feelings when the family member is still ill.

This is likely to be owing to a message we got as children that it was selfish to think of our own needs and wants. This kind of guilt is very common when the person with dementia is put into institutional care.

Andrea Gillies in *Keeper* pokes fun at a serious book on how to be a good carer: 'The Book doesn't seem to want carers to have any sense of relief or liberation when caring comes to an end. That might be unseemly, mightn't it? Being glad. Being glad is taboo.'

Guilt about how we fear others may see us

Guilt can be a cover for feelings of fear. So we may feel guilty if we do something that we worry other people will judge us for, such as putting the person with dementia in a care home. In this case we are focused not on whether or not we have gone against our own values or beliefs, but instead on what we fear other people may think about us. This then falls into the category of inappropriate guilt. We may be afraid of not being liked or approved of by certain people, such as other family members or society at large. If we are closely identified with being 'nice' and 'caring' it may be difficult for us to do something that can be interpreted as tough or assertive.

Guilt when we recognize the 'less nice' parts of ourselves

We all have an idea of the kind of person we feel we 'should' be, and a lot of this self-image comes from the kind of behaviour that was approved of in our families when we were children. These ideas about the kind of person we 'should' be also come from our culture more generally. Among the messages we get from our culture is that it is 'good' to be caring, compassionate, independent, rational and strong. It is 'bad' to be selfish, angry, needy, weak or 'too' emotional.

The more we can accept all the parts of ourselves, the less need we will have to beat ourselves up with inappropriate guilt. When I talk about accepting all these parts of ourselves I don't mean that it is acceptable to act in a way that harms or devalues other people. For example, if an adult daughter grew up feeling that her brothers were treated more favourably than she was by Mum, she may feel some satisfaction if Mum begins to draw away from them and becomes closer to the daughter, who is caring for her. The daughter may feel guilty about these feelings.

But if the daughter, instead of judging herself for taking pleasure in others' misfortunes, can instead accept this part of herself – without feeding the vindictive feelings – and understand it, there is more space for improving her relationship with her brothers. A way of understanding her vindictive feelings may be that there is a part of herself that felt hurt as a child by her perceived unfair treatment and it is this hurt child who is still angry all these years later.

Guilt about lying or breaking promises

You may have lied, or not been entirely truthful, to the family member in order to protect him or her from distress. This is a difficult area, and a 2013 report in the *Daily Telegraph* revealed that two-thirds of psychiatrists and nurses questioned in a survey admitted 'therapeutic lying', or 'white lies', in order not to distress confused dementia patients.

The Alzheimer's Society was reported as criticizing this kind of behaviour by saying that people with dementia should not be encouraged to live in a false reality.

One of the most difficult areas is when the person with dementia asks about loved ones, forgetting they are dead. Reminding her that someone has died can cause a lot of distress for the person with dementia. In an ideal world you would be able to distract her and avoid the dilemma of whether to lie or not.

But if she asks every day, or even several times a day, after her husband, forgetting that he died many years ago, should the carer reply each time that her husband is dead if that leads to anguish and distress?

My feeling is that, although it will depend on the particular situation, it is better to tell a therapeutic lie than subject her to anguish and pain – feelings that may be repeated later in the same day if they need to be 'corrected' again.

I can understand how uncomfortable it might be to withhold the truth from a loved one, but we are dealing here with an unusual situation in which the loved one's mind is degenerating and she is experiencing a different reality. Yanking her out of that reality back to our own world does not feel like the kindest approach.

In any case, you can feel guilty at either approach. If you always tell her the truth you can open up a huge amount of grief and distress or get into an argument that her father, or whoever she is focused on, is really dead even though she insists he is alive. On the other hand, if you go along with the fantasy you can feel guilty about not being truthful. You can't win, really!

Guilt about putting the person with dementia into residential care

Many people feel guilty about putting the person with dementia into a care home. These feelings are natural because we may feel that doing this in some way represents failure on our part. But again, this relates to the inappropriate guilt of not being perfect, not being Superman or Superwoman. In fact, family members are often surprised at how the experience of moving to residential care seems to benefit the person with dementia and actually improves the relationship between him or her and family members.

Former TV presenter Fiona Phillips describes in *Before I Forget* the difficult feelings she experienced when taking the decision that her mother needed to go into a care home. She had tried to come up with a plan in which she could share the caring with her brother, but this would have been impractical given her mother's severe needs:

> I told Auntie Mary [about my plan to look after Mum myself] and she said, 'You can't do that, chick, it'll ruin your marriage, and it's not fair on the children. You've got your lives to think of now.' But I still couldn't help feeling that Mum deserved our care, not the care of strangers, and whatever anyone said, whatever anyone continues to say, I will never rid my system of the guilt.

An adult daughter says:

> Mum had always been extremely self-reliant and had made me promise her I'd never put her in a home, but I got to the stage where I felt I had no choice. I felt guilty about this, but we had a better relationship when we weren't living together any more and I wasn't having to tell her what to eat or what to do, which would always lead to arguments.

What we can do about guilty feelings

The most important thing we can do is be kind to ourselves and tell ourselves we are doing the best we can and that it is all right not to be perfect.

As John Suchet says of the Admiral Nurse who supported him in caring for his wife:

> He taught me that I am allowed to have an off day, that I am allowed to lose my temper, that my behaviour – unusual, even bizarre, though it may appear to me – is normal. I have learned that there is nothing a carer wants to hear more than that the way they are behaving is normal.

When it comes to healthy guilt there are clear things we can do. Healthy guilt is when we have done something specific that contradicts our personal ethics. So, if we lose our temper with the person with dementia and shout at him or her, this will probably offend our beliefs and judgements around treating others with respect. Or if we find that we have been spending so much time on the person with dementia that we have neglected our relationship with a spouse or children, again that is a sign that life has become unbalanced.

To deal with healthy guilt:

- admit what you have done wrong to the person concerned and apologize;
- do what you need to do to stop behaving in the same way again;
- move on.

Healthy guilt is a sign that we need to change our behaviour. Sometimes it will take numerous incidents of feeling guilty over the same behaviour before we are in a place where we are willing or able to change.

Dealing with inappropriate guilt

There will almost always be some inappropriate guilt that we feel, so we need to get used to it but not let it dominate our lives. What this means is allowing the inappropriate guilt to be there but also making a space for a kinder part of ourselves to be heard.

Asking ourselves what the inappropriate guilt may be covering over can be useful. For example, is our guilt covering over anger at someone, such as the person with dementia? Is the guilt a way for us to avoid accepting the legitimate, but less pleasant, parts of ourselves? Or could the inappropriate guilt be a way of keeping ourselves stuck in childhood messages that we need to be perfect or to keep everyone else happy?

By questioning what may be underneath the inappropriate guilt we can then address this underlying issue. This may mean finding a way of honouring our anger, accepting all the different parts of ourselves or allowing ourselves to be imperfect.

You can begin to become more sceptical about your feelings of guilt. You can question whether it is a healthy guilt which is trying to point you in a direction of personal growth. Or you may decide it is inappropriate guilt, which is not there to teach you anything but instead relates to old messages from childhood about having to be perfect, having to put your own needs to one side or having to please everyone else.

8

Shame and stigma

Dementia carries stigma for many people and can lead to a feeling of shame. This applies both to the people with dementia and, by extension, to their close family members.

Stigma

This is linked to shame and is something which causes a person to be 'judged by others in an undesirable rejected stereotype', according to the charity Alzheimer's Disease International (ADI). The *Oxford English Dictionary* describes it as a 'mark of disgrace'. Stigma prevents people from acknowledging symptoms and accessing services for dementia. Stigma is one of the causes of shame and it can make looking after a loved one with dementia even harder.

The *World Alzheimer Report 2012: Overcoming the stigma of dementia* points out that family members and carers of people with dementia may experience 'stigma by association':

> Families face many problems including being afraid to bring memory loss issues to the attention of the person who has them. Moreover, some of the symptoms of the middle stages of dementia, such as agitation and incontinence, inappropriate clothes or dishevelment, can be embarrassing to family members, who isolate themselves and the relative with dementia to avoid having to expose themselves to the reactions they anticipate from those outside the family.

Part of this reluctance to interact with the wider community may be that some of the symptoms of dementia, such as poor self-care and incontinence, could be seen as evidence of neglect.

Shame

What is shame? Its roots come from the word 'to cover' and there is something about shame that is about covering over something, hiding something. In the past people with mental illness or brain disorders were often hidden away from society. Their families felt shame because the message they got from their society was that mental impairments were a sign of weakness or something 'wrong' within the family.

Shame is a very powerful emotion but one that is relevant to dementia because dementia highlights the things in our society that most of us do not want to face – ageing, death, mental deterioration, madness.

In some way this historical shame and fear around madness and people who 'lose their minds' still has a hold over many people, even if they are not fully aware of it.

There is a lot of shame around dementia in our society. This is partly linked to the historical shame that families felt about having a child or relative who was mentally disabled or impaired. But it is also about the fact that someone with dementia is an uncomfortable reminder of things many of us try to avoid thinking about, such as illness, mental decline and death. The fear of having dementia is regarded as worse than cancer, heart disease, diabetes or a stroke, according to a US survey carried out by Harris Interactive in 2011.

Dementia is viewed as cancer once was

The shame and stigma which is now associated with dementia used to be linked to cancer. It was not until the 1970s that patients were told that they had a cancer diagnosis. Before that they were often not told, on the basis that they would be better off not knowing because it was a disease whose cause was not known and which had no cure. Doctors believed that people with cancer would have a better remaining quality of life if they did not know.

Dementia challenges the values of our society

As a society we are almost addicted to busyness – the underlying message we get from many politicians, the media and advertisements is that to be valuable members of society we should work hard and, when not working, consume.

We get messages from the media about what is valuable. Among these are youth, beauty, intelligence, money and possessions. A person with dementia is a living example of everything that is opposite to these values, and that is unsettling for us.

In fact, many of us use our busyness as a way of avoiding thinking about the less comfortable questions – what are our lives for? Are we really happy? The French philosopher Blaise Pascale summed this up in his statement: 'All of humanity's problems stem from man's inability to sit quietly in a room alone.' This culture of always doing something has been challenged in recent years by the popularity of mindfulness meditation, which promotes the idea that it is only by taking a step back from our constant busyness and activity that we can find a deeper sense of peace.

The message that the media gives us is that we can all stay young and healthy indefinitely, as long as we exercise enough and have the right diet or cosmetic surgeon. We may know, rationally, that this kind of message is bogus, but often at a deeper level we take it in and it becomes part of our view of the world and how things should be.

Even when we allow ourselves to consider our ageing and mortality, many of us have bought into the idea, perhaps unconsciously, that we will grow old gracefully, become part of the 'silver surfer' generation, and die a 'good death' surrounded by family and friends.

Dementia also challenges the idea that is embedded in our society of constant improvements and progress. Our cars get better, our TVs are bigger and there is constantly technological innovation. We have cures for many diseases that in the past were deadly and widespread. But dementia is incurable. Like death, the relentlessness of dementia taps into our deep-seated fear of no longer existing.

Perhaps this is why we may feel shame about telling others our relative has dementia – why dementia has become as difficult to talk about as cancer was a generation ago.

Many people with dementia experience shame – they try to hide their memory loss or loss of other functions. They may feel the illness is some kind of reflection on themselves. In one study in Australia, 60 per cent of people said they would feel a sense of shame if they received a diagnosis of dementia and nearly half said they would feel humiliation. In another Australian study, from 2011, 22 per cent of people said they would feel uncomfortable spending time with a person with dementia.

There seems to be something shameful, in our society, in losing one's cognitive functions. For example, we praise older people with phrases such as 'His brain's as good as ever!' We recommend crosswords or brainteasers as ways of keeping the brain healthy – implying that those people whose brains decay bear some of the responsibility.

The medical profession can be part of the problem

This subtle message that there is something shameful about dementia can be reinforced by medical professionals, many of whom seem to completely overlook the person's dementia or to treat the individual in a disrespectful way.

Margaret

I go to medical appointments with Mum and it's hard when the staff just talk to me and ignore her. I know Mum gets confused but it does seem disrespectful. They almost turn their back on her, when they're talking to me.

This reluctance to genuinely acknowledge dementia from both health professionals and people in general can reinforce the carer's belief that there is something to be ashamed of in having dementia, or in the stigma by association, in looking after a loved one with the illness This in turn can make it harder for the carer to feel comfortable accessing services, both for him or herself and for the person with dementia, and can maintain the feeling of isolation.

In the 2012 survey by Alzheimer's Disease International, 11 per cent of carers said they tried to hide the fact that their loved one had received a dementia diagnosis. Some said they did this because the person with dementia was embarrassed about it, others because they felt some shame themselves. When asked if looking after a family member with dementia had led to them being treated differently by others, 28 per cent of carers said yes. Most of these highlighted social isolation as the main problem, such as not being invited to social events or family gatherings or being contacted by friends.

Some carers said that other people could feel awkward around them and not know what to say.

Nearly a quarter of carers said that they had stopped themselves from having close relationships since the dementia diagnosis. Many said they did not have the time or that it was too hard to maintain relationships in the face of the kind of demands placed on them by looking after the person with dementia. Others highlighted what they perceived as a widespread lack of understanding from others about dementia and the burden it places on family members.

The impact of shame and stigma

One of the effects of experiencing stigma and shame is that the carers or family of the person with dementia may be more likely to hide or downplay what is going on. This can mean a delay in diagnosis or accessing services. It can also lead to increased social isolation.

Shame and stigma in some minority communities

Shame and stigma can be particularly acute in some minority ethnic communities, such as south Asian families. In many south Asian languages there is no word for dementia, except for 'madness'. Families can feel a lot of shame if one of their members develops dementia and this can stop them from seeking a diagnosis or accessing services.

Fatima, an outreach worker who works with families of south Asian heritage in London, says:

> The culture is that the family looks after its own and there is a fear that the children's marriage prospects will be affected if people outside the family know about it.
>
> In some south Asian communities dementia is not seen as an illness or brain disorder but as an indication of the sins you've committed. I know one Pakistani woman who took her mother to access dementia services and was shunned by the local community and seen as a bad child because she wasn't doing everything herself for her mother. Often an older person with dementia who is in a traditional south Asian family can be left sitting all day in their armchair, with no stimulation, and then they go downhill fast.

9

Coping with loss and grief

> There is no life without loss and therefore no life without grief.
>
> (Miriam Greenspan, *Healing Through the Dark Emotions*)

In many ways, being a carer for someone with dementia or being closely involved with that person means facing loss. This does not have to be loss of something specific that we used to have, but may also be loss of what we might have had were it not for the dementia.

But one of the major challenges of dementia is that, until the very end, there is not a physical death, which can be grieved, but rather an often long process of change and deterioration. It is like a continuing process of loss but, for long periods, without the finality of physical death.

Peter

Losing my wife before her physical death was very difficult, and there was one particular day when my heart was broken. It was a cold, snowy January day and I found her sitting in our car in the garage, with the doors locked. She wouldn't respond and I couldn't unlock the door, so I ended up having to crawl into the car through the boot to get her out. During that whole process she said nothing. That was the day I knew I'd lost her.

Of course, despite the changes to behaviour, memory and cognitive abilities, the person with dementia is still present and able to be connected with in a meaningful way, even if it is not in the way that we are used to relating to him or her.

Grieving the losses associated with dementia is one of the most important parts of the family carer's experience. But many carers may go through the process without knowing that they are grieving. Being aware that you have experienced major losses, or will be facing them in future, and that these losses need to be mourned is an important part of adapting to the losses.

Once the grief is named it becomes easier to talk about and deal with.

This kind of loss has been described as ambiguous loss and grief, because it is not clear cut but instead is a gradual process in which you may have confused or conflicting feelings about what is happening. While many family carers experience this ambiguous loss and grief, they may not fully recognize what is going on and how to deal with the feelings.

This can leave you feeling confused and in a kind of limbo – unsure of whether or how to grieve the losses that have occurred or are currently occurring, and also aware of the losses that are still to come.

In some ways coping with the loss and grief associated with dementia can be more stressful and complex than actually providing care.

Different kinds of loss

There are numerous losses that may be felt.

- *The gradual loss of the person with dementia.* She is changing, losing her 'old self', dying.
- *The death of the person with dementia.*
- *The giving up of your job or familiar life.* You may have had to give up or reduce your work, have moved house or made other major changes in your life.
- *The loss of your old identity.* You may feel you are giving up your role as spouse or (adult) child, to become a carer.
- *The loss of other relationships or interests.* Dealing with the person with dementia may squeeze out, or make impossible, the continuation of certain other relationships or interests.
- *The loss of intimacy and companionship with the person with dementia.*
- *Financial losses.*
- *The loss of what might have been.* That is, expectations and hopes for yourself or for the relationship with the person with dementia.

There is also the loss of the self. It is not just the person with dementia who can experience a loss of the self, but also the person looking after him or her. Because caring for someone with dementia can become such a dominant part of your life and all the focus seems to be on him, you can sometimes feel that your personality has become subservient to his.

Sadness and grief are the ways that we deal with losses in our lives. Both these emotions, even though they may feel uncomfortable or painful, are a necessary part of healing. This is important to recognize – that sadness and grief are not just painful or 'negative' feelings that we should avoid or suppress. They are essential experiences that actually help us come to terms with losses and, ultimately, move on with our lives.

By 'moving on' I don't mean that we somehow no longer feel any pain or sadness, but rather that the pain or sadness around the loss is less acute and we are able to adjust to the loss. In terms of dementia, experiencing and working through grief enables us to adjust to the changing relationship with the person with dementia.

In early stages grief can sometimes be difficult to recognize because it can show itself in numerous ways.

Some symptoms of grief include:

- feelings of hopelessness and despair
- guilt
- sadness
- social withdrawal
- anger and frustration
- lack of concentration
- physical aches and pains
- insomnia, lack of appetite, lowered immunity.

Differences in grief reactions between adult children and spouses

Spouses or partners may experience grief differently from the adult child of a person with dementia. For example, studies have shown that on average grief increases significantly for spouses when the person with dementia moves into a care home, but not for adult children. Adult children, on the other hand, are more likely to experience anger and frustration as part of the grief process.

Adult children are also more likely than spouses to have social support, which helps them cope with grief. A particular problem for many spouses is when they have relied on their partner for socializing and, now that the partner has dementia, they find themselves feeling even more isolated because the 'sociable' partner is no longer active.

Sadness

You cannot protect yourself from sadness, without protecting yourself from happiness.

(Jonathan Safran Foer, US novelist)

Humans need to experience sadness. It helps us cope with loss and disappointment. But many people see sadness as 'negative' and try to avoid feeling it, perhaps afraid that if they allow themselves to feel it they may sink ever lower.

This is nearly always a mistaken fear, as often people feel better after 'a good cry'. They may have taken in the message that it is self-indulgent to allow oneself to feel sadness. With all the suffering in the world, we may tell ourselves that life isn't too bad, so allowing ourselves to feel sad can seem selfish.

Or we may rationalize our reluctance to acknowledge sadness by telling ourselves that it won't change anything, so what's the point?

But sadness is a healthy emotion to feel when we are in pain. In fact, it can help us get through that pain – whether it be a loss we are experiencing, an awareness of someone else's pain or sometimes just a vague sense of something missing.

Difference between sadness or grief and depression

There is a difference between sadness or grief and depression, although there is clearly also an overlap between the two. Usually sadness has a fullness, an aliveness to it. It may be painful but we may also recognize that, at a deeper level, it is life-affirming because it is connecting us with our vulnerability, our longings and fears. Depression, on the other hand, often has a dryness and a deadness about it.

Sadness can help us connect with others, for instance if they see our tears. Depression often isolates us from others, leaving us feeling lonely and cut off.

A clue that shows the difference is that there is often a lowering of self-esteem involved in depression.

The value of tears

One of the most common indications of sadness is tears. Although there are also tears of frustration or even joy, crying usually communicates sorrow to others.

We may feel embarrassed or uncomfortable crying in the presence of another, particularly in our culture where 'too much' emotion is viewed as undignified. But sometimes we cannot control when or where our tears come to the surface.

Unlike 'reflex' tears, which allow our eyes to get rid of harmful particles, emotional tears contain stress hormones that leave the body when we cry, thus reducing stressful feelings. In addition, when we cry it stimulates our body to generate endorphins, which are natural pain and stress fighters.

Crying also has a powerful psychological benefit in enabling us to express difficult feelings. Crying does not necessarily solve our problems, but it does mean the feelings of sadness are no longer just inside us – they have been given a healthy outlet.

The benefit of crying may depend on the context, however. So if you cry somewhere public and feel embarrassed or shamed because you think you are being judged, then the stress benefits of crying may be outweighed by the discomfort of feeling embarrassed.

Grief is a natural emotion

Like sadness, grief is a normal emotional response. It is a deep or intense sorrow we feel when we experience a major loss, especially the death of someone who is, or has been, important to us. But it can also be applied to other major losses. Mourning is the process that one goes through when adjusting to the loss.

Grieving is a natural human emotion. It is also something that animals do, with grief symptoms having been reported in cats, dolphins, geese, elephants and many other species. In a famous study by Konrad Lorenz, a greylag goose that had lost its partner was found to show all the symptoms that psychologist John Bowlby observed among young children who were separated from their parents.

Although there may be stages or tasks involved in grieving (see page 68), grief is not a linear process. There is no time when one is 'over' the loss; rather, there is a coming and going of sadness, with more intensity at certain times. Gradually the sadness, or other feelings, will lessen but there will still be times when difficult feelings return, although usually in a more manageable way.

The process can be even more challenging because we live in a largely secular society in which the traditional role of religion has diminished. Lacking these old certainties can make knowing how to grieve more difficult.

But because dementia is a slow decline and death, it is accompanied by a complicated grieving process.

Disenfranchised grief

Disenfranchised grief refers to losses that are not generally recognized by society as needing to be grieved. This may include divorce, the loss of a pet or a miscarriage. It can also include the kind of losses experienced by someone caring for a loved one with dementia. Disenfranchised grief is when the person grieving gets the message that he or she does not have the 'right' to grieve a particular loss.

As well as the fact that we do not experience the finality of a physical death and the opportunity to grieve that death, we do not experience the same level of support from family and friends as we would if a loved one had actually died. If someone close to us dies, people around us recognize that we are going through a grieving process, but the nature of loss and grieving in dementia is much less obvious to others.

We may get the message from people around us, or from society at large, that we do not need to grieve or that we are spending too long in the grief process. The message communicated may be 'Stop feeling sorry for yourself.'

Because others may not understand what we are going through, and we may not even understand it ourselves, we can feel alone and isolated with our grief. Friends and even family members may not understand why we feel grief, as they have not experienced the changes in the relationship with the person with dementia. They may not appreciate the huge losses we are experiencing – in the dreams and aspirations we may have had for ourselves or for our relationship, or in other losses such as sacrifices in our professional life or in other interests and relationships.

Ambiguous and anticipatory grief

As we have seen, ambiguous loss and grief refers to the psychological loss that carers may experience. It is called 'ambiguous' because the person with dementia is still alive and therefore there is no physical loss, but he may not be mentally or emotionally present in the same way as he used to. This may be experienced as a major loss for the family carer.

Anticipatory mourning means experiencing grief in anticipation of the losses that are likely to occur. This can occur throughout the progress of the illness. According to the Alzheimer's Society, there is some evidence that carers who experience anticipatory grief cope better with the grieving process when the person with dementia actually dies.

Part of the difficulty with grief and dementia is that because the illness can last many years there may never seem an appropriate time to really acknowledge the grief. In the early stages it can seem wrong to talk about, or even think about, the death of the person with dementia, because it seems a long way away.

There is also the fact that the decline involved in dementia is not completely linear. Someone's memory may come and go; there will be good days and bad ones. This can mean it is sometimes hard to grieve a final loss when there may be the possibility of apparently lost faculties returning.

Margaret
My father died of a brain tumour and that was very difficult but at least it was final, there was some closure. With Mum's dementia it's about loving someone who is gradually disappearing, and that's heart-breaking.

The whole nature of dementia can make grieving extremely complicated. If the loved one has changed and no longer remembers the same things or behaves in the same way as in the past, does this mean she is a different person? Who has she become? Is there a core self that is always there, even if we cannot see it?

You may also be so preoccupied with the practical challenges of caring for or helping the person with dementia that deeper, uncomfortable emotions such as grief are for much of the time not consciously felt.

Frozen grief

When grief isn't acknowledged or expressed it can become 'frozen' – it is there but it is not being consciously experienced. Frozen grief can have a damaging effect on a person – in terms of physical ailments, stress or depression.

Grieving takes time

For anyone grieving, but particularly for someone close to a person with dementia, the grief process takes time. Whether it is grief over the gradual losses associated with the disease, grief over a move into a care home or grief over the physical death of the loved one, the process happens in its own time and cannot be rushed.

Just as for someone grieving a loved one who has died, significant dates can be important in the grieving process for a still-living loved one with dementia. These can include Christmas, birthdays, wedding anniversaries and so on. It is often on these days that you will be more in touch with the losses that you have experienced.

'I try not to dwell on sadness and I've got used to never getting any more birthday or Christmas presents from John,' says Susan, a phlegmatic carer for her husband.

You may be surprised at how suddenly grief can surface as dates such as these approach, so it is important to allow yourself to feel the feelings and not judge yourself as weak or as not coping.

Give yourself permission to grieve

Because we usually associate grief with a physical death, it may not seem right to have these feelings when the loved one is still alive, even though we know that we have experienced major loss. We may feel it is not respectful to the person with dementia for us to acknowledge to ourselves, let alone express to others, our feelings of grief over what has been lost.

But, even though it sounds counter-intuitive, allowing ourselves to feel the pain of the loss is what helps us come to terms with and – eventually – move on from the loss. The alternative is to deny the loss to ourselves, to keep busy, to try to keep permanently cheerful. But this does not deal with the loss, it just builds up a deeper reservoir of pain that is not visible from the surface but is present nevertheless and influencing our emotional state.

It can sometimes happen that we feel so overcome by the pain of grief that we suppress it and instead express an emotion that helps us feel more in control, such as anger. So, when the person with dementia can no longer remember significant things or people, instead of allowing ourselves to feel the sadness and grief, we may find ourselves feeling irritated with him or her.

It is understandable to feel some frustration when the person with dementia behaves in unusual ways or can't remember what seem to us like obvious things. But when we get angry, even though we know that the forgetfulness is a part of the disease and not deliberate, we may be covering over the vulnerability we feel at knowing our loved one's brain is dying and that this death is irreversible.

People have different ways of grieving

Different people have different styles of grieving. There is a 'feeling' style, in which you feel waves of strong emotion, and moving forward involves exploring and expressing feelings. This approach, which is more common among women, is sometimes known as an 'intuitive' style of grieving.

There is also a 'doing' approach to grief, sometimes known as an 'instrumental' style of grieving. This involves more thinking and less overt feeling – there may be an inward, quiet process and less visible expression of emotion. This approach, which is more common among men, values doing something active, finding out information that will help, analysing ways forward.

While these styles may be seen as in some ways 'masculine' or 'feminine', this is just a generalization and there will be men who grieve in a 'feeling' way and women who grieve in a 'doing' way.

Those with a 'doing' style of grieving may appear to be further down the line of handling their grief, because it seems less visible. This may not be the case, however.

Neither of these approaches is 'right' or 'wrong' and many of us will adopt a mix of the two. If someone, whether a man or a woman, does not feel at all comfortable talking about sad feelings to a group, then there is little point trying to force it. That only leaves the grieving person feeling stigmatized and uncomfortable.

On the other hand, sometimes people with a 'doing' style may benefit from being encouraged to talk about their feelings but this should only be done if they are receptive to the idea.

What carers need is being allowed to grieve in the way that feels most appropriate for them and in their own time. At the end of this chapter there are some suggestions of ways to deal with grief which are relevant to both 'feeling' and 'doing' styles.

Common triggers for grief include:

- when symptoms are noticed;
- diagnosis;
- when the person can no longer be left alone;
- loss of driver's licence;
- loss of shared memories, e.g. holidays;
- move to a care home;
- when the person no longer recognizes key people, including the carer.

When the person with dementia actually dies

You may think that when the person with dementia actually dies, often after a long decline, the feelings of grief will be less because you have already been through much of the grieving process. This is not necessarily the case and you may be surprised by the strength of emotion you feel.

Also, the emotions you feel when your loved one actually dies may be mixed. There may be a part of you that feels relief that she is finally 'out of her misery' or that you no longer have to spend half your life worrying about her.

The tasks of mourning

One way of looking at the grief process is as a series of tasks that need to be completed in order to come to terms with the loss. Bereavement specialist William Worden describes these in his book *Grief Counselling and Grief Therapy*. The concept of tasks that need to be undertaken gives the griever a more active role than the earlier concept of phases of grief, which suggests a more passive experience for the griever.

Of course, grieving can be a complicated process, particularly the ambiguous and anticipatory grief experienced by the family carer. While the grieving process cannot be rushed, the idea of certain tasks that need to be completed can give the griever a feeling of personal agency and help him or her feel a little less helpless.

Below are the tasks of mourning. Although they are in a certain order, the process of working through the tasks is not necessarily linear and you may experience more than one at the same time. Also, tasks may be revisited and worked on at different times. The tasks are focused on a physical death, but are also relevant to the grief you may be experiencing concerning the losses experienced in caring for a person with dementia. The tasks are:

- accepting the reality of the loss;
- working through the pain of the grief;
- adjusting to a new environment;
- emotionally relocating the deceased and moving on with life.

1 Accepting the reality of the loss

This is the first step in the grief process. Unless and until you accept that you have experienced a major loss you are not able to mourn that loss. When someone dies, the loss is more obvious than the smaller and more subtle losses that a family carer of someone with dementia experiences. But nevertheless, the losses experienced by the carer are real and need to be recognized.

One way of not accepting the reality of the loss is to deny it or minimize it. So, you may tell yourself that the loved one's loss of memory capacity is temporary or that his or her memory is not as bad as it seems and that it may return. Or if you've had to give up your job to care, you may tell yourself you didn't particularly like that job anyway and so it's not a big loss.

Often family carers can be so focused on the practicalities of looking after the person with dementia, organizing everything, planning ahead, that the experience of loss and of grief can be smothered.

2 Working through the pain of grief

Society can be uncomfortable with grief, either the ambiguous grief described above or the more 'normal' grief following the death of the person with dementia. You may get the message that you should not spend 'too long' grieving or that you should be grateful that the person with dementia is finally out of his or her misery. This can combine with your own mixed feelings about the death – a part of you feeling relief, perhaps, that this long, painful saga is over and another part of you grieving the final loss of your loved one.

The most common way of avoiding this task is by not feeling the feelings. This can happen through denial or downplaying the loss, by distracting yourself with busyness and practicalities or by trying too hard to stay 'positive'.

3 Adjusting to a new environment

In Worden's model, this refers to a new environment in which the deceased is missing. In the case of dementia, however, the loved one may still be alive even though important aspects of his or her personality or of the relationship are missing or have changed significantly.

For you it may mean adjusting to the loss of your role or identity in some way. So, you may feel you are no longer that person's lover, or child, in quite the same way as in the past. Instead of him doing all the driving and maintaining the car, now he is no longer able to fulfil that role. Or you may have relied on the person with dementia to do all the cooking or housework, so need to adjust to the new reality.

You may feel some resentment at having to learn new skills that were previously performed by your partner. But, in time, you may come to feel some satisfaction at acquiring new skills and experiences that you had previously ruled out for yourself because they were in your partner's domain.

The adjustment may also be to an internal change in self-identity. So instead of seeing yourself as this person's spouse, lover, companion, you may begin to see yourself more as his or her carer, although these different identities will be mixed together.

Part of adjusting to a new environment is what Worden calls a spiritual adjustment. This is about finding, or searching for, meaning in the losses and the life changes that accompany them. The losses involved in caring for someone with dementia can challenge your view of the world. If you have viewed the world as at heart a benign place, having to care for a loved one with dementia can bring up issues of anger and a sense that the world is unfair and random.

4 Emotionally relocating the deceased and moving on with life

This may be the most difficult task, and particularly so for someone whose loved one has dementia and who is coping with ambiguous loss. It is about finding a way to stay connected with the person who has died, while being able to re-engage with life. In the context of dementia that may mean finding ways of remembering the person we knew, while staying in relationship with the person undergoing the changes brought about by dementia. It is about making a place in our emotional life for the person who has been 'lost'. This may be achieved through our memories, speaking to the 'lost' person or through dreams. It may be through recognizing that person's values that we have taken on in our own life.

Some ways of working through grief

Below are some ideas about how to handle grief. Some of these may work for you and others may not. It is also important to acknowledge that the nature of caring for someone with dementia will have practical implications for some of these ideas – if you are not able to leave your loved one alone for more than an hour, or at all, it will be difficult to find the chance to walk in the countryside, for example.

Talk to someone

Others around us may not appreciate the level of loss and grief we may be going through, and we may not fully realize it ourselves. That means we can downplay our feelings to ourselves, suppress them or believe that they are 'wrong'.

Recognizing that they are a normal part of looking after a loved one with dementia can help us to accept these feelings. In itself, acceptance of feelings is a powerful first step to dealing with them.

Talking to someone who understands – or can truly empathize with – what we are experiencing can help us feel less alone and more 'normal'. That person may be a friend or relative who has gone through a similar experience or is knowledgeable about our situation, or it may be a counsellor, support group or dementia helpline or internet forum. The 'Useful addresses' section provides contact details of some of these.

Seeking support can also provide you with strategies for how to cope, especially if you are talking to someone who has been through the same experience.

Do something physical

For some people, doing something physical can help handle feelings around loss. This may be jogging, chopping wood or going for a long walk in the countryside.

Doing something physical that has some personal meaning, in the context of the person with dementia, can also be therapeutic. For example, if it is your spouse who has dementia and she always wanted a white picket fence at the front of the house, taking action to make that fence a reality can be a very personal way of channelling grief feelings into an activity that is meaningful.

Writing

- Write a letter to the person with dementia, expressing your thoughts and feelings. You can then find a way to ritually dispose of the letter – perhaps tearing it up and throwing the pieces into the sea, or burying the pieces at the base of a new plant.
- Write a blog.
- Write a poem.

Anticipate difficult dates

Thinking ahead and anticipating difficult feelings around anniversaries, Christmas or other holidays can help reduce the stresses at those times.

Stay in the present moment

While it is important to make a place for sadness over what has been lost, it is also important to stay in the present and appreciate what is there. Even though the person with dementia may have lost the ability to remember or communicate important things, meaningful connections are still possible. Time spent doing something simple, such as holding his or her hand or speaking in a kind way, can be meaningful for both of you.

Part 2
RELATIONSHIPS

10

Family tensions

When a member of the family has dementia this can bring up wider issues within the family. In some ways the effect on the family can be positive, as having someone who needs care and attention may lead to the family uniting and pulling together. In other cases, however, the stress of looking after the person with dementia can highlight existing tensions and bring new ones.

The way that different members of a family get on with each other – or fail to get on – has been established long before the person with dementia becomes ill. But these relationship patterns will have a major impact on how the family handles the challenge. If, for example, the adult children of the person with dementia have had a difficult relationship with the parent in the past, that will impact on whether and how they involve themselves with providing support and care.

There may be tensions between siblings about who is doing more and whether the person with dementia is being supported in the right way. Of course, when everyone is feeling tired and overwhelmed by the demands of dealing with dementia, tensions and disagreements are more likely to come to the surface.

Often one member of the family will end up taking the majority of the caring responsibilities, and this can lead to resentment towards other relatives who are perceived by the carer as not doing their fair share. The reason one particular child or relative becomes the main carer may be geographical, or it may be because he or she has fewer other commitments, such as a demanding job or children.

In some cases the adult child who takes on the main carer role may feel he or she has a different relationship with the parent from that of the siblings, such as feeling closer.

Daughters as carers

When it comes to adult children, it is often (but by no means always) one of the daughters who takes the main carer role. This is because, despite some cultural changes in perceptions of male and female roles, caring is usually still seen as primarily a female quality. Historically, it was sometimes regarded as the youngest daughter's role, or that of the daughter who remained unmarried, to look after the parents in their old age.

These beliefs still live on in many families, with the result that it is often the adult daughter who takes on the lion's share of the caring responsibilities. This is not just true of dementia but also of caring more generally.

Margaret

The caring for Mum has largely fallen on me, helped by my sisters. I have several brothers and I know if I rang any of them up to say a shelf needed putting up they'd be round, but they don't see her that much. Maybe that's because they don't know how to handle her in this state. I'm not sure they really appreciate her condition in the same way that I do because I see her all the time.

In an article about caring for her mother, who has cancer, novelist Claudia Carroll bemoans the praise heaped by her mother on one of her brothers for visiting, even though he lives much closer to the care home than Claudia and has visited far less.

I'm certainly not complaining about my [caring] duties. This is just what you do if you're a half-decent daughter and your mother is unwell . . .

I'd be worried sick if I wasn't here to keep an eye on her. But I simply can't help noticing that my mother's illness doesn't seem to have affected my two brothers in the same way it has me.

While her brothers phone regularly, they seem to be relatively unaffected by their mother's illness. One of the hardest things for her is that her brothers' visits seem to generate such pleasure for Mum, even though she, the daughter, feels she has had to take on much more of the day-to-day responsibility for Mum.

You only have to look around Mum's ward to see that, by and large, women are those who support their elderly parents. Daughters – especially the single ones – are expected to assume the role of nurse and carer, while sons can observe from a safe distance.

Relatives who live at a distance

Another potential problem that can arise when there is a main carer living with or near the person with dementia and other siblings living further away is that the non-local relatives may not appreciate the severity of the situation. Because they are not seeing the person with dementia on a regular or sustained basis, siblings living far away can tell themselves that the parent is not in such a bad way as the main carer says.

What can reinforce this view is that people with dementia are often able to perk up and put on their best face when there are visitors. So the brother or sister visiting for a few hours may see a perkier, more competent version of the person with dementia than is the reality.

Aislin
I feel exasperated sometimes at my brother and sister. They both live a long way away, while I'm close to Mum, and I don't think they always see things like I do. My brother will visit and Mum will put on a special effort – he's her only son and they've always had a good relationship so she rallies a bit when he's there. But I think he's been in denial about how serious her condition is. Likewise, when Mum visited my sister abroad she managed to adapt quite well, but it's very different dealing with her at home on a daily basis – I see a very different picture.

Areas of disagreement

Here are some of the key decisions that families can disagree about.

- Is there actually a problem? Initially, some family members may be adamant that Mum or Dad is just a bit forgetful or depressed.
- Should the person with dementia be assessed? When is the right time?
- What should happen over financial matters?
- Who should do the main caring?
- Where should the person with dementia live?
- Should the person with dementia be put in residential care? When is the right time?

Positive family relationships

But as well as cases where the adult child who becomes the main carer feels resentful towards siblings, there are also situations where other brothers and sisters are able to help. An adult child who is taking on too much may be supported by siblings and helped not to take on more than is appropriate.

Tensions between the adult child and the non-ill parent

When one parent has dementia there may be tensions between the adult child, or children, and the non-ill parent. These tensions will be fuelled, in part, by how these relationships have developed previous to the illness.

For example, the husband of a woman with dementia may not be willing to accept what is happening and may instead feel resentful that his wife is no longer behaving in the same way she used to.

Writing in the magazine of the AARP, the American retired people's organization, Alex Witchel describes how her father refused to move on from his view of her mother as the woman who looked after him whatever he needed. This was despite her developing dementia. Over the phone he would complain to his daughter that her mother kept getting his breakfast wrong, which he saw as a lack of attention rather than a symptom of dementia.

> My siblings and I looked to our father for guidance about Mum's situation but he wasn't giving any. For the 50-plus years of their marriage, he had considered her the superwoman/wife/mum. She took care of their children, and she took care of him. The idea that he take care of her seemed to confound him.

This kind of behaviour is often extremely annoying for the adult child, who does not know if he or she can really trust the non-ill parent to take care of the person with dementia. Behind the apparent callousness, however, may be a huge fear on the part of the non-ill parent. He may be afraid that if he genuinely allows in the information that his spouse has dementia it could be too over-whelming (see Chapter 2 on denial).

Fernanda

My mum developed signs of dementia in her late 60s, but we didn't recognize it at first because she's always been a bit difficult – emotionally distant, obsessive. But when she started forgetting about doctors' appointments we thought there was something wrong.

One major challenge has been that she won't accept help – she doesn't even like to accept that she actually has dementia even though the diagnosis was a year ago. She won't take the medication she's been given and won't let carers in.

All this has brought family tensions to the fore – it's me, my sister and brother, and we've never been that close, but things have got worse with the pressure of my mum's dementia. My sister and I tend to agree on most things concerning Mum's care, but my brother often disagrees. He was against us getting the diagnosis and he said he'd organize getting a power of attorney, but he never got round to it.

There are tensions between the three of us about who is doing the most to support Mum, who is feeling most stressed and so on. I feel resentful that my brother doesn't seem to do as much as me and my sister.

The family arguments have been one of the hardest parts of Mum's dementia and it's something I wasn't really expecting. It would be nice to have a united front, but we seem to relapse into childhood sibling rivalries and arguments.

Mum needs someone to accompany her to doctors' and hospital appointments and that is often me. My brother won't do it even though he's single and has more time.

Having said all that, I wonder if the three of us siblings would be in touch at all if it weren't for Mum's illness. At least we've had to talk to each other about how to support Mum, even though there are often annoyances that boil over.

11

The nature of the relationship

The nature of the relationship you have had with the person with dementia will have a big impact on the kind of emotions you experience and how you handle them. It will also impact on the experience of the person with dementia. The well-being of the carer and the quality of the relationship between carer and cared-for have been found to have a significant impact on when the person with dementia moves to a care home.

Research carried out in the 1990s by US researcher Lore K. Wright suggested that low levels of interaction between the partners in relationships where one person had dementia predicted entry to institutional care and even the death of the person with dementia within two years.

Therefore, the higher the level of stress the person in the caring role is under, the more strained the relationship is likely to be. One of the biggest problems, particularly in spousal relationships, is the loss of intimacy.

If you are a spouse or an adult child of a person with dementia there will probably be many factors from the past that will influence how you feel and behave towards this person. Some of these factors you will be aware of but some are likely to be less conscious.

Some research suggests that many spouses report more areas of satisfaction when it comes to caring than do adult children. A report by Jan Oyebode in the journal *Advances in Psychiatric Treatment* (*APT*) says that the emotional investment of spouses may lead them to feel more involved, less burdened and less likely to seek a care home for the person with dementia than are adult children. There are contradictions in the research, however, with another study suggesting that partners of people with dementia are more likely to experience depression.

There are also sex and gender differences in the behaviour of men and women with dementia, which can impact on the relationship with the carer. According to research on men and women with Alzheimer's, cited in Sally-Marie Bamford's report *Women and Dementia – Not Forgotten*, men more commonly demonstrate verbal incoherence, apathy and excessive sleeping, as well as aggressive behaviour, including sexual aggression.

Women were more likely to show reclusive behaviour and intense mood changes, with behaviours such as hoarding, refusing help and inappropriate laughter and crying. The report pointed out, however, that there are divergent opinions on the link between sexual aggression and men, with the possibility that sexual behaviour by men is more likely to be judged negatively, while similar behaviour by women may be overlooked more easily or may lead to a protective response by carers or families.

The majority of those caring for people with dementia are women. For example, one study from Canada, quoted in *Women and Dementia*, found that three-quarters of carers for people with dementia in the community were female, as well as 71 per cent of carers in health or social care settings. But there is evidence that when it comes to caring for one's spouse, men and women are almost equally likely to be providing care.

Ambivalence

The psychological term 'ambivalence' can help us understand something about our relationships with loved ones. Ambivalence is when we have conflicting feelings towards a person, often at the same time, and that inner conflict can cause us unease or discomfort. Some degree of ambivalence is present in all close relationships. It can be quite freeing to know this because otherwise we can easily judge ourselves. Difficulties in accepting ambivalent feelings can lead to intense guilt and anxiety on the part of the carer. We may say to ourselves, 'I shouldn't be feeling angry with my mother – I love her!' Or, 'I feel so much care and affection for my husband, but I also feel as if I hate him sometimes – what's wrong with me?'

Ambivalence is a normal part of any close relationship, and when it comes to being close to someone who has dementia it is even more likely to be present. This is because the illness puts great pressure on close relationships, especially when the person we thought we knew begins to behave in very different – and often difficult – ways.

One of the clues that a person is not recognizing these ambivalent feelings is when he or she makes sweeping, idealized statements about the relationship or the other person. These may include, 'We have always had a perfect relationship, with never a cross word,' or 'She was the perfect mother.'

The more we can accept the different, and sometimes contradictory, feelings we have towards the loved one, the more at ease we will be with him or her. Some of us are very identified with particular roles or feelings and may see ourselves as 'a loving son' or 'a caring wife'. That can mean that we reject any possibility of feeling unloving or uncaring towards this person.

But it is completely normal for us to feel unloving or uncaring at times, and to feel anger or even hatred in the moment. That does not make us a bad person. These are only feelings. The danger in this situation is that we are trying to be too perfect. By not allowing ourselves to accept the part of ourselves that can feel 'negative' feelings, we end up repressing those feelings, which means that at an unconscious level we push them away and pretend to ourselves that they are not really there.

This repression requires a lot of energy, making it actually harder for us to be kind, loving and caring – all the things we want to be. In addition, the difficult feelings do not just disappear but can make themselves felt in less conscious – but damaging – ways.

If we reject or disown parts of ourselves – such as our angry or selfish parts – we can end up projecting these emotions or energies onto the other person. This is something we do without being conscious of it, but it can be very damaging to a relationship.

Adult children

Daughters are more likely than sons to feel a sense of obligation to provide care and take on the caring role, according to the *APT* report. For those daughters who have their own children there is particular strain. There may also be the stress of combining work commitments with a caring role. But marriage can help buffer daughters from strain, with those who are married reporting they receive more support and experience less depression than those with no partner.

Daughters may report more distress in caring than spouses, the journal reports: 'This is possibly because many spouses have already reduced the number of other commitments in their lives and may have expected to care for their partner, whereas daughters experience greater disruption to their lives to accommodate the caring role.'

The most obvious is a feeling of obligation, duty or love. Your parents brought you into this world and, mostly, looked after you as best they could given their own experience of being looked after by their own parents or caregivers. This feeling of obligation will encourage you to look after your parent now that he or she needs you, or someone close, to provide care.

But relationships with our parents are usually more complicated than this and many of us will have more ambivalent, or mixed, feelings. Alongside the feelings of love and duty there will be other feelings, depending on how you experienced him or her as a parent when you were a child. If, for example, you at times felt rejected or not loved or respected as a child, you will have more mixed feelings towards this person, even if the predominant feeling is one of love or kindness.

It can be incredibly frustrating experiencing the transformation in the relationship with a parent when you become his or her carer. It is as though you have stopped being the child and become simply the carer. This frustration may be worse if you had a difficult relationship with that parent when you were a child.

Likewise, the experience of becoming a carer for your parent will be particularly difficult if you had a difficult relationship with your parent when you were younger, or if you had an extremely close relationship with that person. It may seem obvious why 'losing' a parent you felt amazingly close to should be hard. But why if you had a difficult relationship?

This is because, if we are carrying resentment from that early relationship, even if we are not fully aware of it, that resentment will have an effect on our current emotions. We may also, at a deeper emotional level, want to 'put right' a relationship that still troubles us. For example, Marianne Talbot, in *Keeping Mum*, describes how her brothers were always her mother's favourites while she felt a little in their shadow. She wonders if becoming Mum's carer was, in part, motivated by the desire to feel important to Mum as an adult because she didn't feel this as a child.

Spouses and partners

Research has thrown up differences between the way many men and women experience caring for their partners who have dementia. According to studies cited in the *APT* report, women report greater stress than men and also report more behavioural and emotional challenges of a husband with dementia, compared with husbands caring for a wife with dementia. It is possible, however, that men caring for a partner with dementia may play down or be less aware of their stress because that is how they feel they are expected to be.

One study suggested that husbands were actually more anxious than wives, perhaps because becoming a carer was a much less familiar role than for many women. A study by couple relationships therapist John Gottman, quoted in Terrence Real's book *How Can I Get Through to You?*, suggested that even when men appeared outwardly unaffected, if they were experiencing distress or conflict their hearts beat faster and their bodies produced more adrenaline than those of their wives.

Although this research has not been replicated by other researchers, it does suggest that the differences between how men and women feel emotion may be less clear cut than some believe. One possibility may be that men are not brought up to value their emotions and so become used to suppressing them or distracting themselves from difficult feelings.

In the *APT* report there was evidence that husbands were more likely to say they felt satisfaction in being a carer than were wives. Many husbands said they felt they were able to repay some of the care they felt they had received from their wives in the rest of their relationship. In contrast, many wives who had devoted a large part of their lives to caring for a family were more likely to say they felt resentful at again finding themselves in the role of carer.

In terms of the caring style of husbands and wives, the research suggests that men are more likely to take a task-oriented approach and be more emotionally detached. They were also more likely to get support from family and health or social services. But over time the feeling of burden that many wives felt was found to reduce and become more similar to that felt by husbands. This may be due to wives gradually becoming more task oriented and less emotionally involved over the period of caring.

As with adult children who become carers, if the spouse had an excessively close relationship with the person pre dementia, or a particularly problematic relationship, then the experience of becoming a carer will be even harder. Andrew Balfour, writing in *Looking into Later Life*, says: 'Those [partners] most at risk are those who have had the poorest relationships [before the dementia] . . . but also those who have experienced the greatest sense of loss of intimacy as a consequence of the disease.'

12

Identification with the carer role

A carer is a person of any age, who provides unpaid support to a partner or relative, who couldn't manage to live independently or whose health or wellbeing would deteriorate without this help.

(The Royal College of General Practitioners)

Becoming a carer involves loss

When you find yourself in the role of carer without asking for it, you are also losing, or giving up, a lot. You may have had to move to a different part of the country to look after the person with dementia, often giving up your social network and support.

You may also be giving up other identities or, at least, shifting your sense of who you are. For example, if you have to give up work or reduce it you may experience a changed status in the eyes of society – those who are paid to do a job generally have more status than those who look after others without pay.

In a sense, as a carer you absorb the values of the society you live in, which in our case values money, possessions and what we produce and consume far more than the willingness to look after other people.

You may find that you no longer quite feel like a lover or spouse or partner because the other person does not share the same memories or relate to you in the same way as in the past. Thus, you have had to give up certain other roles or identities.

If the person with dementia is no longer able to communicate effectively with others, you may feel that in some way it is now your responsibility to maintain his or her identity. There is frequently some irony to this because, in becoming a carer, your own identity will often have shifted significantly if you have had to give up work or other interests.

Are you the 'family caretaker'?

Many of us have roles assigned to us within our families from when we are children, although we become so used to these roles that we do not realize we have them. These roles can include the 'super achiever' or the 'scapegoat'. One of these roles, usually assigned to a girl, is of the 'family caretaker' – the child whose job is to take care of others' needs at the expense of her own. The family caretaking child may have one or both parents who are depressed, addicted or emotionally wounded in some other way, and so she remains bright and cheerful to keep them happy.

Family caretakers often take jobs in the caring professions, such as nurses, social workers or therapists.

Some people who end up as carers for a parent or spouse with dementia have always been the family caretaker. An important thing to realize is that one of the reasons the family caretaker looks after others is to gain some good feelings about herself. Anyone who has taken on a rigid family role as a child has not really been seen and accepted for him or herself. People in this position have not genuinely had their needs met. Therefore, there is frequently a shaky sense of self-esteem at the heart of the family caretaker.

By taking care of others the family caretaker gets to feel positive about herself, but unfortunately the caretaking does not really address the deeper problem. The family caretaker is good at taking care of others but not so good at acknowledging her own needs and getting those met. Family caretakers often feel extremely guilty that they are not doing enough, even though everyone around them tells them they are doing more than enough.

Because family caretakers are either not aware of, or don't value highly, their own needs, they find it very difficult to ask for help.

Margaret

I'm the eldest daughter of ten children and I've always been like the family's second mother. Since I was six or seven I was helping Mum by changing the younger ones' nappies, helping with cooking and cleaning.

Since Mum has had dementia I've taken the lead in looking after her, along with my sisters. I find it very difficult to separate emotionally from her when I'm not with her so I worry about her all the time. The only time I don't is when I know she's with one of my sisters.

My husband's mother has MS so I'm often juggling helping my mum and mother-in-law and trying to help everyone stay in good spirits. It's hard for me sometimes because I don't like to ask for help.

Do you play the rescuer role?

The 'rescuer' role is linked to the family caretaker role. Chapter 13, on the drama triangle, describes how many family carers gravitate towards this 'rescuer' role. People who are attracted to the rescuer role are often eldest or only children, or grew up in chaotic families. They often learned that they could avoid conflict or trouble in the family by being 'good'.

The rescuer has a lot of rules about how he or she should behave and what other people want. But it can be very tiring constantly working out what others want and trying to give them this, so the rescuer can easily feel like a martyr and risks exhaustion.

Rescuers also find it hard to know what they themselves want, because they can be so focused on what everyone else wants.

Having to be perfect

While there is some helpfulness in the word 'carer' I believe that there are problems as well. One is that if you are a carer, then what about your own needs? If your role in life is caring for someone else, this implies that your own wants and needs are less important.

It also implies that you should be this perfect, thoughtful, helpful, 'caring' person, when you might not feel that way. So, when you find yourself feeling angry with the person with dementia you may beat yourself up – 'If I was genuinely caring, I wouldn't feel like this,' you might say.

But unless you give yourself permission to feel angry, resentful or fed up you will be less able to genuinely care. Allowing yourself to feel these emotions is not the same as expressing them to the person with dementia. It may be that you need to find a safe way of expressing them, such as to a friend or family member you trust.

The Shadow of being a carer

We all have a Shadow. This psychological term was invented by Carl Jung to describe the parts of ourselves that we repress, hide or deny. We repress or hide these parts of ourselves usually because we do not like them or they do not fit the image we want to show the world. So they tend to include our selfish, greedy, deceitful, arrogant or cruel parts.

But the less aware we are of our Shadow, the more it controls us and brings us problems. For example, if we deny the importance of getting our needs met, by regarding this as 'selfishness', we push our selfishness into our Shadow and will probably then end up projecting this onto others. The result is that we then see selfishness in others all around us and we judge them harshly.

Particular roles can also have Shadows. The Shadow of the carer role may include selfishness, being controlling and self-importance.

Although carers generally have low status in our culture, there can still be a subtle attraction in the role for some people. At least it means that you are needed by someone and therefore that you are important.

In itself I don't see this as a problem. It is natural to want to feel wanted or needed. But it is problematic if this is part of the attraction for us of being a carer and we don't acknowledge it to ourselves. We may not want to acknowledge it because it does not fit in with our image of ourselves as caring and altruistic. But whatever we repress about ourselves comes out in other ways, usually negative.

By taking on this identity of 'carer' you may, in some way, become persuaded that only you can provide the right kind of care for the loved one. For example, a carer may go away on holiday for a break while relatives look after the person with dementia. When the carer is told, on returning, that the person with dementia has seemed surprisingly happy in his absence the carer can feel a tinge of disappointment. What he really wants to hear – or at least a part of him wants to hear – is that the person with dementia has seemed sad but has perked up now that the carer is back.

It is this feeling of 'I'm indispensable' that can prevent carers from taking breaks, but this can make the whole caring experience more stressful for both parties. It can also delay the move of the person with dementia into a care home.

Sometimes carers are surprised by how much happier the person with dementia is when he or she moves into a care home, particularly if the relationship between the two people has become tense and strained in the run-up to this.

It can seem unfair that you, the one who does the most for the person with dementia, can sometimes seem to have the most difficult relationship with her. All kinds of tensions can come to the surface, such as feeling jealous and resentful when she seems to be so pleased to see your brothers or sisters, who don't do half as much for her as you do.

The move into a care home

The idea of moving the person with dementia into a care home can bring up many, sometimes conflicting, feelings. These can include guilt, fear and even relief. There may also be anger at the financial wrangling with the statutory sector that can accompany this decision.

Keith

There's a real problem around working out when it is appropriate for the person to go into a care home. With my mum, we'd ask social services and they'd say it was very difficult to predict. She was getting a lot worse, so I asked in February and social services said she'd probably need to move by September. She ended up being moved much earlier, in May, and in a very rushed way just after I returned from holiday to find she had got a lot worse.

The problem is, the funding comes out of the social services budget, which is constantly being cut. I know the local authority is in a difficult situation, but they could be more supportive and anticipatory because otherwise all the stress falls onto the family.

In the event, I lied to Mum about what was happening, telling her it was a respite break. This was because she'd been saying she didn't want to go into a home. I felt a bit guilty about this but she actually settled in fairly quickly and hasn't mentioned not wanting to be there at all.

For many of us, we have internalized the message that old people are better off being looked after in their own homes, almost no matter how complicated their needs are. This message can be reinforced by a financially strained system that wants to put off taking people in until the last possible moment.

Politicians do not always play a constructive role in this debate, with some coming out with comments praising south Asian immigrant communities' ethos of taking care of their elderly, and implying that Western families are somehow aiming to get their relatives institutionalized as soon as possible.

This kind of lecturing from (usually male) politicians does a disservice to the commitment of family carers, many of whom have made huge sacrifices to look after or support their loved one. It also completely fails to highlight the pressures on families caused by the economic structures that we all live under – the fact that in many families both parents need to go out to work.

But this kind of contribution from politicians feeds into an assumption that people are better off at home, as do the media stories about poor treatment of residents in some care homes.

The need to let go

Sometimes you may end up trying to keep your loved one out of a care home even though it is in his or her best interests. This can be for a variety of reasons. For example, the process of finding the right home can be time consuming, or there may be complicated financial issues to deal with.

But it can also be the case that you have got so used to looking after someone that you cannot imagine anyone else doing this job. It is not uncommon for the carer to lose perspective because she is in the middle of this exhausting situation. Often it is only a few months later that she can see how close she was to breaking point.

Cora
I felt guilty putting Mum in the care home, but I felt like I had no choice. Once she was there we got on a lot better and I could be her daughter again rather than her carer – I wasn't having to tell her what to eat, what to do any more and having to get into arguments.

There comes a time when you need to let go of being a hands-on carer. This is the point when the needs of the person with dementia have become too complex and demanding for you. It may also be the case that the closeness of the relationship, all the shared history and baggage, is actually not working in his or her interests.

'Giving up' the person with dementia to a care home may feel like a betrayal, but sometimes part of this is our own desire to remain indispensable, valued, needed.

Claire

My mum wouldn't take the medication she was prescribed and the GP said there was nothing we could do except to wait for a crisis. I found her in bed after Christmas in her own excrement, confused and dehydrated. I called for an ambulance and she went to hospital, where she picked up infections.

I told the hospital that no way could she return home, and when I said I'd rent out her home to pay towards care home fees the local authority were happy. Before she entered the care home there were times when she was very aggressive towards me, but since she entered the care home we've got on the best we've ever done, partly because she is now taking her medication. She still recognizes me and seems glad to see me. I sometimes feel guilty that she's not still in her own home but she's doubly incontinent and she wouldn't accept carers in the house, so it would be almost impossible.

13

The drama triangle

One way of looking at how relationships can go wrong is the drama triangle. This applies to many different kinds of relationship, including romantic relationships, family relationships or work relationships. I think it can also shed light on the relationship between a family carer and the person with dementia.

The drama triangle (Figure 1) was developed by US psychiatrist Stephen Karpman in the late 1960s.

In this model there are three roles that are played – persecutor, victim and rescuer.

The persecutor is the person who bullies or hurts and the victim is the person who feels hurt or bullied. Perhaps the most interesting role, and the one that is usually hardest to understand at first, is the rescuer. This is the person who 'knows best', who can be rather superior, who advises and who has 'nice guy control'.

Many carers fit most easily into the rescuer role. It is a role they are familiar with. It helps them feel important, needed and in charge. The rescuer hates to feel like a victim – after all, part of the

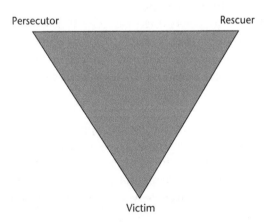

Figure 1 The drama triangle

rescuer role is to deny one's own needs and vulnerabilities. As a result, when you are in rescuer mode you are likely to project your own vulnerability and anger onto the person with dementia. You feel extremely uncomfortable with these feelings, so it is much easier to see them in the other person while you continue to be 'nice', 'caring' and 'sensible'.

We do not usually realize that we are in one of these roles, as this is mostly happening at an unconscious or semi-conscious level. We are particularly unlikely to acknowledge it to ourselves if we are being the persecutor, as this may not fit in with our image of ourselves as being caring. Likewise, we may not like to see ourselves as the victim if we prefer to see ourselves as strong and independent.

We move between roles

It is important to recognize that the people in the relationship move between these three roles, constantly changing the pattern of the relationship. However, one or both people may tend to gravitate towards one of the roles more of the time.

In the moment the drama triangle is being enacted there is always someone 'on top', who seems to have more power, and someone who feels like the underdog. This can change, as roles change, so that the person who felt on top now feels at the bottom.

When spending time with the person with dementia you may find yourself moving between these three roles at different times of the day, or even within the same hour.

The fact that many carers often gravitate to the rescuer role can actually cause more problems than it solves. When the carer tells the person with dementia to do something in an 'I know best' fashion, it can trigger rebellion. This, in turn, can leave the carer feeling like a victim.

Or the carer, in the rescuer role, can feel unappreciated – 'Why am I doing all this and not getting any appreciation?' he may ask. At this point the carer may shift into the persecutor role by having a go at the person with dementia, often over something trivial. The message to the person with dementia may be something like, 'Why do I have to do everything? Why can't you show some appreciation? It's so unfair!'

In a sense the person with dementia is a genuine victim – a

victim of the illness and of the progressive lack of capacity it brings. But the carer can also feel like a victim – having to give up work, hobbies, time, money, friends, in order to help the person with dementia.

Power imbalances

The drama triangle shows up power imbalances in relationships. While on the surface you may be the one with the power in your relationship with the person with dementia, it is not actually as simple as this, as you have probably found out. Yes, you can make the big decisions but your loved one can wear you down, refuse to co-operate or adopt any number of strategies that leave you feeling like a victim and powerless.

The fact that he or she may be cognitively impaired makes this model a little more complex, but I believe it is still relevant. Unlike in some other relationships, with a person with dementia it may at times be necessary to 'rescue' because he or she cannot realistically be allowed to make certain decisions or engage in certain behaviour, such as driving.

But if you prevent her from driving, because you believe she is not safe to do so, you may be felt to be a persecutor and she may feel like the victim. She may then get angry with you, leaving you feeling like the victim and her the persecutor.

Sometimes you may find yourself running around trying to get something sorted out for the person with dementia, only for her to turn round and not want it. You are in rescuer mode but she may be feeling pressured or controlled, so to stay with some feeling of power she refuses what you are offering.

The important thing in this kind of situation is to recognize that you have stepped into a particular role and then ask yourself if you really need to be in that role.

Being part of the drama triangle is not a good place to be – not good for you and not good for the person with dementia. This is because we gravitate to these roles as a way of avoiding uncomfortable feelings. For example, we may be in rescuer mode as a way of avoiding feeling our fear about the future or our sadness about the present – it is easier to take action, to get something practical achieved, than to just acknowledge our feelings.

How to get out of the drama triangle

The first step is recognizing when we are in it! The more we can see that we have been drawn into the role of rescuer, persecutor or victim, the more choices we have about how to respond.

We can then choose to go to our 'adult' part. This is the part of us that can take responsibility for what we are feeling, rather than automatically blaming others. It is the part of us that can take a step back from our behaviour, thoughts and feelings and observe them in a more detached way.

When we notice we are in one of the three roles, we can allow ourselves to simply take a step back, rather than automatically continuing in that role. If, like many family carers, we gravitate towards the rescuer role, it can feel uncaring or callous to step out of that role, but the reality is that when we do this we become more vulnerable, more human. And this will be picked up by the person with dementia, who may recognize that we are not seeing him or her as someone to 'rescue' but as someone with specific complex and conflicting needs who may need a bit more space.

It may be worth asking yourself if that thing you are telling your loved one to do is really essential – is it life or death? If not, then a suggestion is fine but then, leave it up to him or her.

Likewise, if the person with dementia is feeling sad or depressed, can you allow him his feelings instead of desperately trying to cheer him up? Or if you believe his diet could be better, can you allow him to make his own decision rather than insisting he eats healthily or manipulating his diet – which often ends up with him going to the victim role.

14

The inner child and other sub-personalities

Many of us see ourselves as coherent, unified individuals making our way through life. But, when we really think about it, we may recognize that actually we are made up of many different parts which come into play in particular situations and which sometimes seem to take over our normal personalities.

These 'sub-personalities' can play a very important role in our lives without us realizing. The more aware we can become of them, the more fully we can live our lives and be present in relationships. Hal and Sidra Stone, in their book *Embracing Our Selves*, explore the different kinds of sub-personalities.

Being aware of these different parts of ourselves can help us in our role as carer. This is because if we reject certain parts of ourselves, or sub-personalities, we drive those energies into the unconscious where they become more powerful and operate beyond our control.

When they are in the unconscious we are more likely to act out destructive feelings, such as rage, or to experience burn-out or illness.

Many of you will be very comfortable with certain parts of yourself – the part that is caring, the part that is responsible, that is logical or sensible. But there will almost certainly be other parts, other sub-personalities, that you feel much less comfortable about, or may even be unaware of. These are the parts that were disapproved of when you were a child and that you now reject within yourself, or that our culture disapproves of.

For example, if we have been brought up to be 'nice', 'caring' and 'hardworking', we will have the opposite energies within ourselves, although we may not like these or even be aware of them. These may include an 'inner idler', an 'inner bully' and an 'inner taker', who surface in certain situations – perhaps when we are under stress or under the influence of alcohol.

Our disowned selves

These are the parts of us that, usually as children, we learned were not acceptable to our parents or others around us. In order to be loved, we then disowned these parts and pretended to ourselves we did not have them.

These disowned parts become part of what psychologist Carl Jung called our Shadow, as we saw in Chapter 12.

How do we discover our disowned parts?

The biggest clue to what parts of ourselves we have disowned is the people we judge most harshly. It is the people who really get to us, who press our buttons. Often we feel some pleasure at judging these people, a certain self-righteousness. This is because what we have unconsciously disowned within ourselves, we project onto others and judge.

So, if we get really annoyed by people we perceive to be selfish, that is a clue that we have disowned our own selfish part. Or we may really get irritated by people we judge to be self-important or self-regarding – again, this is a clue that we have a disowned part that is like that.

Dreams also tell us about our disowned selves, often represented by intruders trying to break into our house, or wild animals that pursue us.

Most people's sub-personalities include:

- *The inner child* – this is our feeling self, the part of us that can be vulnerable, afraid, playful, joyful, angry.
- *The protector or controller, our 'ego'* – this is who we think we are, the part that watches over us, that tries to control our environment. It is a bit like our inner parent.
- *The pusher* – the part of us that tells us we must get on and get stuff done and holds a whip over us. There is never enough time for everything that needs to be accomplished. The pusher's list of things to do is endless. When we are having a break, it is the voice that reminds us of all the things that still need attention. The pusher is linked to the inner critic sub-personality.
- *The perfectionist* – like the pusher, the perfectionist is often linked to the inner critic. The perfectionist is the part that insists any-

thing we do must be perfect. Something that others would regard as 'good enough' is regarded as shoddy and embarrassing by the perfectionist.

- *The pleaser* – this is the part of us that always wants to do the 'right thing' so that others are happy. It is the part of us that is always available to others, always there to help, that rarely thinks of our own needs and wants.

The aware ego

We can also develop what Hal and Sidra Stone call an 'aware ego' – this is the part of us that can observe ourselves, that can witness. It can be developed through mindfulness or simply by noticing what we are thinking and feeling without judgement. When we can be in our aware ego, we can take a step back from the protector–controller, which is the part of us that worries about what others will think of us, which always has a goal in mind and thinks it is rational.

In becoming more aware of the different parts of ourselves, by developing the aware ego, we can come to accept ourselves more. The process is about accepting all these different parts of ourselves rather than judging them.

So, to avoid our inner bully acting out we need to find a way of honouring our natural anger or aggression because the inner bully becomes more powerful the less we are able to accept our angry part.

Honouring does not necessarily mean expressing the anger, although there will probably be times when we do express it in the moment. But honouring may mean simply being aware of our anger and finding a way of giving it a place in our life. That could mean talking to someone about our feelings, writing about them, reading poetry, doing something physical like hitting a pillow with a tennis racket, and so on. There is also a process called voice dialogue, in which you have a 'conversation' with the disowned part, which the Stones describe in their book.

By becoming more aware of what we are doing, of the behaviour of the different sub-personalities, we are able to consciously choose what we want more easily. So, for example, instead of automatically giving and giving until we are exhausted, we can choose whether, and how, to give.

One of the most important sub-personalities is the inner critic, which I cover in Chapter 15.

The inner child

Another of the most important sub-personalities is the inner child. This represents our vulnerability, fear, playfulness and creativity.

Many of us, and particularly many family carers, bury this part of themselves because they tend to be identified with looking after others and meeting others' needs.

In the context of looking after someone with dementia, you may often feel as though you are a parent looking after a child. This can reinforce the disowning of that child part of yourself.

Because parents often unintentionally squash the spontaneity and vulnerability of the child, we can take on their attitude and identify too much with our inner parent, which can be represented by the inner critic or the protector–controller.

It is important for us to acknowledge our inner child and to honour it, but not to let it run our lives. If you find yourself feeling frequently irritable, exhausted or tense, that's a sign that your inner child needs attention.

Your inner child may need:

- more sleep;
- more play;
- more opportunities to be creative;
- less pressure from the inner critic;
- more quiet time or time for oneself.

Looking after the inner child, not indulging it

It is up to us to acknowledge what our inner child is feeling and find ways of helping it gets its needs met. This is not the same thing as letting the inner child rule our lives, in the same way that we don't let any single sub-personality take over.

For example, we are creating problems if we try and quieten our inner child's longing for attention or love by giving it alcohol, inappropriate sex or high-risk activities, or if we let it run riot with temper tantrums.

A more healthy response is finding ways to acknowledge, or feel, the feelings and to reflect on appropriate responses to the inner child's needs and wants.

More details on how to get to know your inner child and how to respond to its needs can be found in *Recovery of Your Inner Child* by Lucia Capacchione.

15

The inner critic

One of the most powerful, and potentially destructive, sub-personalities is the inner critic, and many carers have a highly developed critical voice in their head that tells them they are not doing enough or are not good enough. We may experience this critical voice as a thought or we may not be conscious of it at all because it has become so much a part of us.

But if we pay attention to our thoughts we can begin to hear what the inner critic is saying. It may say:

'I shouldn't feel angry. If I feel angry I must be a bad person.'
'I can't believe I made that mistake – I'm just not good enough.'
'I should be able to handle any situation with ease and good humour – if I can't there's something wrong with me.'
'If I feel sad that means I'm weak and I must always be strong and in control.'
'I'm a terrible daughter/son/husband/wife.'
'I don't deserve to take time off for myself – that's just selfishness.'

The origins of the inner critic

The inner critic often takes up residence in our heads as a child and it frequently sounds like one of our parents or some other important adult. The inner critic represents the critical side of that person, so even if in many other respects he or she treated us well, if he had certain high standards or expectations, we may absorb that part of him until it becomes a part of us.

The inner critic is the voice of the parent (or other significant adult) when he or she was most rejecting or annoyed. We then carry around that critical voice without realizing it – but it can make our lives a misery.

Imagine the inner critic's voice as like an endless loop of cassette recordings in your head, telling you the same negative things again and again.

The inner critic is linked to the inner perfectionist – the part of us that tells us we must be perfect or we will not be loved or acceptable.

Often the inner critic uses words like 'should', 'ought' and 'must'. It tells you that you 'should be more understanding', you 'ought to feel less irritated' or that you 'must try harder'. This kind of language is usually not helpful and we can use it as a stick to beat ourselves with. But most of us use these words all the time without realizing it.

When we notice ourselves using 'should', 'ought' or 'must', we can pause. Often it is more helpful to say 'could' instead of 'should'.

The inner critic's message is directed at the child part of us – the inner child. It is an internal drama – like a parent scolding a child, except that it is happening inside our minds.

You can never please the inner critic

It is important to recognize that you can never do enough for the inner critic. Whatever you do, it will find a way of putting you down.

How to handle your inner critic

The first step in dealing with your inner critic is to externalize it. By this I mean imagining that it is a character with its own personality. What does it look like? Is it male or female? What is the tone of its voice? What is its name?

By giving it a name and a character you no longer see the inner critic's comments as simply 'you', but rather as a distinct part of yourself. Gaining some distance between 'you' and the inner critic makes it easier to handle because you now know what you are up against.

To get a sense of what your inner critic is like, begin to notice what it says. Then allow yourself to imagine what it looks like – is it a big, looming dark presence? Or a short-tempered school teacher with a cane? Or a skinny, purse-lipped middle-aged woman?

Next give it a name that sums up its character – 'Brenda the Bully', 'the Sergeant Major', 'the Judge'.

By giving it a name and a character you weaken its power and become more able to recognize when it is talking.

The value of mindfulness

One of the best ways of dealing with the inner critic is with mindfulness. What is mindfulness? Well, mindfulness courses and mindfulness-based cognitive therapy, have become very popular in recent years. Derived from Buddhist meditation and some cognitive behavioural techniques, the courses are aimed at helping people live calmer, less stressed lives.

Essentially, mindfulness is about paying attention to what is happening in the present moment: just observing it without judging. To develop this present-moment awareness you can follow your breath or become aware of your body.

The idea is that by following your breath or becoming aware of the physical sensations in your body, you detach from the constant chatter of thoughts and judgements in your head. With the help of the focus on the breath or body you can instead begin to observe this chatter without becoming entangled with it.

When it comes to the inner critic, mindfulness helps because the best way of combating the critical voice is simply observing it. Trying to argue with the inner critic doesn't work because this simply gives it more power. You cannot beat the inner critic by rational argument.

What the inner critic hates is being ignored. So, if you become aware that the inner critic is running you down about something, you can simply notice this and take your awareness to your breath or your body. The more you can practise this, the less powerful the inner critic will become. Remember, the inner critic is not simply going to disappear because you argue back, but over time it will become less vocal the more you can ignore it.

Becoming more mindful can help you get more in touch with your bodily sensations, which can provide clues about the activity of the inner critic. It may be indicated by a tightening of the jaw, a constriction in the chest area or a heaviness in the shoulders.

Mindfulness and emotions

Mindfulness is also very useful for dealing with difficult emotions. This is because, instead of trying to get rid of feelings of sadness, fear or anger, we can learn to experience them without feeling we need to do something about them – to get rid of them, distract ourselves or act them out.

Mindfulness is about breathing into what we are experiencing – not pushing it away, but not fanning the flames either. It is simply noticing what we are experiencing.

So many of our difficulties with emotions come from our emotions about the emotions. In other words, the problem isn't that we feel sad or anxious or angry, because everyone feels those emotions from time to time. The problem is when we feel there is something wrong with us for feeling what we are feeling, that we are weak or a failure or a bad person if we feel certain feelings. For more details about mindfulness, see *The Mindful Way Through Depression*, by Mark Williams and others.

16

Empathy and not taking it personally

Empathy is what you can bring to the relationship with the person with dementia. It can help both of you have a less antagonistic, more meaningful relationship.

By empathy I don't mean feeling sorry for the other person, but rather an ability or willingness to enter into her world a little, to imagine what life feels like for her and to allow that knowledge to shape your responses.

Alongside empathy, it can be very valuable to have an attitude of not taking things personally. When someone with whom we have had a deep and sometimes complicated relationship develops dementia it can bring up a lot of difficult feelings inside us. We may at times feel criticized or attacked, or we may feel unappreciated or misunderstood. It can be automatic to take this behaviour personally, but we don't need to do that.

Not taking the behaviour personally

When we feel criticized or disrespected by the person with dementia, it is natural for us to feel angry, sad or hurt. He may show no appreciation for all our efforts; he may seem completely oblivious to how annoying his behaviour is; he may even be accusing us of stealing from him or betraying him in some way.

The problem is not the feeling itself – that we feel hurt or angry – but taking the behaviour personally even when it feels very personal. Can we allow ourselves to feel our anger or hurt, while at the same time recognizing that the loved one's behaviour is to do with the dementia?

Because we will have a shared history, and usually plenty of baggage, with our loved one it can be easy for us to take things personally. When people with dementia enter a care home, frequently their condition improves because they are being looked after by people who don't have that personal, historic connection and therefore are able to not take things so personally.

A carers' support group worker says: 'A lot of carers see the person with dementia as being devious – that word comes up a lot. They interpret the person's behaviour as a deliberate attempt to give the carer a hard time.'

When we are able to not take the loved one's behaviour so personally, we are able to take a step back and see his or her behaviour in a different way. We can see it as having its own reasons and meaning, even if that meaning may not be immediately clear.

How we treat someone influences how he or she behaves

Many of us know that if you treat someone in a certain way, he or she will often begin to behave in that way. If a child gets the message that she is 'naughty', she will often end up behaving in that way because that is how she begins to see herself.

In the context of dementia, campaigner Tom Kitwood in the 1990s promoted the idea of 'malignant social psychology'. By this he meant that the negative way dementia is viewed in our society and the negative way people with dementia are treated actually affects the progression of the disease.

The way we view and treat the person with dementia has a big effect on how he or she feels and on the relationship. The more we can metaphorically stand alongside someone and imagine her world, the more she will feel accepted and understood. If we judge her, tell her that her behaviour is ridiculous or driving us up the wall, she is far more likely to feel vulnerable and emotionally unsafe.

Of course, we are human and we may sometimes show our exasperation, anger or distress. But when that becomes a habitual response to difficult behaviour there can be problems.

Empathy and time

One of the big differences between those with dementia and those without is the experience of time. For most of us in our busy lives, time is rather like a commodity – it is something we often feel we don't have enough of, that we'd like more of. We measure time and often evaluate whether we are spending our time efficiently or productively.

This is particularly true in northern Europe; it is perhaps a little less so the further south you travel, and in many traditional cultures time is experienced in a much freer, more flexible way.

Someone with dementia will probably have a very different experience because he or she will not have the familiar reference points of the past or a firm conception of the future – everything is in the present moment.

This can cause huge frustrations for you, accustomed as you are to time being precious, to things needing to be done by a certain time, to the awareness of the consequences of taking 'too long'.

Making sense of unusual behaviour

If you are a close family member or friend you will probably know something of the history of the person with dementia, and this can be important because it can help make sense of her actions and feelings. It can help you to be sensitive towards her when she is no longer able to express her thoughts and feelings.

For example, if the person with dementia suddenly becomes anxious at a loud rumbling noise, you may be able to link it with the fact that as a child she experienced the bombing in the Second World War. Making that link to the person may help her feel in some way understood and therefore lessen her anxiety.

The loss of language and cognition experienced in dementia also means that the person may be communicating what he is feeling and experiencing in a symbolic way or through his behaviour. A carer who is empathic and who knows something of the person's history may be able to make sense of what seems, on the surface, to be simply disruptive or inexplicable behaviour.

In her book *Looking into Later Life* Rachael Davenhill, a psychoanalyst, tells the story of a woman with moderate dementia in a care home, who is moved into a unit occupied by those in a much more advanced state of the disease. When a newspaper in the room is removed the woman becomes anxious and angry. Her anger and distress seems inexplicable, but Davenhill speculates that the newspaper symbolized the outside world and connected her to her earlier life of no mental deterioration. The sudden disappearance of the newspaper represents her imprisonment in mental decline.

One lens through which we can look at dementia is attachment theory. This was developed by the British psychologist John Bowlby, who studied how children reacted when separated from their parents. The theory looks at how humans feel and behave when separated from parents or primary caregivers, known as 'attachment figures'. Bowlby believed that this pattern of seeking attachments to caregivers was part of an evolutionary drive to increase the chances of survival.

Attachment theory argues that for the child to grow up as confident, feeling loved and able to regulate its feelings, it needs to have a secure attachment figure, such as a loving and reliable parent or primary caregiver. If a child lacks a secure attachment it may grow up to feel either too needy or too independent, and will find it hard to trust in adult relationships.

Clingy behaviour

While attachment theory has primarily focused on infants, it can also have relevance for people with dementia. They experience huge changes in their relationships to loved ones (attachment figures), caused by the deterioration of their brains, and this leads to increased levels of insecurity and anxiety. Not only are they are less able to rely on these relationships because of the disease, but also they experience the disease getting progressively worse. Bowlby found that when the child experiences the threat of losing the attachment figure, it can become clingy and seek closeness.

This kind of behaviour is a common experience for carers and those close to people with dementia. They often report how the person with dementia can follow them round the house, not want them out of sight and so on.

Dutch researcher Bere Miesen carried out studies into this among people with dementia. As well as attachment issues with the spouses or loved ones of people with dementia, he was interested in the 'parent fixation' shown by many people with dementia. This means the belief that one or both parents were still alive even though they were long dead. This is a common occurrence among people with dementia, asking to see or talk to one or both parents and not accepting that the parent is dead.

If we bear in mind the huge fear and insecurity experienced at times by the person with dementia, we can imagine how trying to bring back one's parents could help someone try to achieve some level of calm or reassurance.

In attachment theory it is not the parent's ability to always meet the demands of the child that is most important, but rather the parent's sensitivity to the emotional state of the child, the ability or willingness to imagine or sense what the child is feeling – in other words, empathy.

This knowledge of how attachment theory is relevant to looking after someone with dementia has profound implications for the relationship between carer and loved one, believes clinical psychologist Andrew Balfour. But he points out that one of the main differences between this relationship and that of a parent and child is that the latter contains a hope for growth and developing relationship, in which the child gradually becomes more independent. That of the carer and the person with dementia, on the other hand, contains the opposite expectation – one in which the cared-for person becomes ever more vulnerable and dependent and which is leading to decline and death.

Jealousy

It is not uncommon for the person with dementia to become very jealous towards his or her partner, suspecting that the partner is having or wanting to have an affair, or that someone else has designs on the partner. There is usually no basis to these fears but the person with dementia can quickly become convinced that he or she is going to be betrayed or abandoned.

Jealousy is a natural part of being human and we have all experienced it to some degree, whether in romantic relationships, in friendships or as a child when we felt a brother or sister was getting more attention or favours from a parent.

According to Freud's Oedipus complex, as small children we want to possess the opposite-sex parent and part of the struggle of early childhood is realizing that we cannot have that parent to ourselves. While Freud focused on the experience of boys, Carl Jung introduced a similar theory for girls, called the Electra complex. It is in learning to negotiate these very strong feelings of desire, possessiveness and jealousy, as well as competitiveness with the same-sex parent, that the foundations for a healthy sexual identity are created.

You do not have to agree with Freud on all this, but it is nevertheless true that many of us, as children, experienced jealousy of a sibling. Even an only child with no other 'competitors' in the household may be jealous of the attention that the parent gives other children. Even though we may feel embarrassed about it, we may as adults find ourselves feeling jealous.

Jealousy in children is a normal feeling. It only becomes a problem if it is judged harshly by adults and so the child gets the message of being unacceptable, of being somehow 'bad'. Because children's capacity to make sense of their feelings is under-developed, they need adults' help to make sense of their experience. If jealousy, or any other strong emotion, can be acknowledged by the parents and talked about in a non-judgemental way, its power will be lessened.

But many children, particularly in earlier generations, will not have had their jealous feelings acknowledged and made sense of. Instead, the feelings – and the pain associated with them – remain unresolved and often repressed.

In dementia, some of these old childhood wounds can return because they never completely went away. The feelings of fear and insecurity stimulated by the illness can be communicated by the person with dementia through jealousy of the spouse.

Feeling stolen from

Another common symptom of dementia is feeling stolen from. Rather like jealousy, this suspicion or paranoia is not simply a random effect of the illness but can be seen as a distorted response to loss. The person with dementia is losing something incredibly important – her mind. Because she is losing her cognitive and reflective ability, it can be difficult for her to be aware of what exactly is happening, but she does know, at a deeper level, that something valuable is being taken away.

This, understandably, can lead to feelings of anger, distress, fear and confusion. One of the ways people with dementia make sense of this loss, and these feelings, is by projecting them onto an actual theft that they imagine has taken place. This can be very distressing for the loved one who is accused of stealing, as no matter how much he protests his innocence he will not be believed.

Aislin, whose mother has dementia and is being cared for primarily by her husband, has been accused of all kinds of 'thefts'.

> In the past 12 months suspicion of me has risen and anytime Mum can't find something – a coaster next to her bed, a tissue – she blames me or my partner for stealing it.
>
> I used to get very upset when this first started and try to justify myself. I'd feel angry and defensive. If I insisted it wasn't me she'd say it must have been my partner who took it. I've got more used to it now and can see that it's not personal or mean, but rather her way of making sense of what's happening to her.
>
> I always had a difficult relationship with her, which is maybe why she accuses me rather than my dad, but I feel sad about it. I've returned my key to their flat and I now only see them outside their home. She recently lost something while I was on holiday and thought it was me but then realized it couldn't have been and that confused her even more.

The carer as 'container'

It can sometimes feel as though you have become the 'container' for the emotional pain that both you and your loved one are going through. It is almost as if you have taken on some of his pain, fear, anger and confusion – emotions that he perhaps is not able to fully understand or experience consciously.

So, you will have your own particular fears, frustrations and confusions but at a deeper level it may be that you are also experiencing some of his, too.

Being a container does not have to be about 'negative' feelings – it can include love and joy. The important thing is about being receptive to what may be being communicated.

Through the psychological concept known as projective identification, someone who is not able or willing to experience certain emotions can induce these emotions in the other person. This may be particularly true in the case of someone, such as an infant or person with dementia, who cannot understand or talk about what may feel a fragmented or confused emotional experience.

In psychoanalytic terms, the other person (the parent of the child or the spouse or adult child of the person with dementia) can become a 'container' for these emotions. By allowing him or herself to experience these emotions, the carer 'contains' them for the person with dementia.

In practical terms what this may mean is that not all of your emotions are actually 'yours', particularly if you are spending a lot of time with someone who is not able to make sense of his or her own emotional life. So, if you find yourself feeling intense anger towards that person, or despair, or love, it can be helpful to tell yourself that some of that emotion may belong to her and not all of it is yours.

Being able to 'contain' that emotion – in other words, not automatically expressing the anger or panicking at the fear, but seeing it as a possible communication from the loved one – can help both of you.

By allowing the possibility that not all of an intense emotion is yours, it can lighten the load for you. And it can also, at a deeper level, affect the person with dementia because, in some way, he or she will feel understood. A good way of handling this situation is saying something to your loved one about what you think may be happening. If you are feeling intense anger or fear, you could say: 'I wonder if you are feeling angry or fearful – that would be very understandable.'

It is about having a curiosity about the feelings of the person with dementia, and not just dismissing them as irrational or inexplicable.

Childlike behaviour

It often appears that the person with dementia at times reverts to a childlike way of being. Meanwhile, the carer, whether that be spouse, adult child or some other family member, can feel like the parent.

This can be very frustrating, and very weird, for you as that person's spouse or child. For the spouse it can change the whole nature of the relationship – from partner or lover to parent – while for the adult child it can be disorienting to find oneself suddenly becoming the parent figure.

This dynamic is not uncommon for some adult children, as through simple ageing the nature of their relationship can change so that they feel they have almost become the parent. It is not for nothing that old age is sometimes described as a 'second childhood', as it brings increased vulnerability and dependence.

But for the adult child or the spouse of a person with dementia there is the added component of the severe deterioration of the brain. This can make completing even apparently simple tasks, such as washing, eating and dressing, very difficult without supervision. Also, the person with dementia may regress to childhood memories, such as calling for Mum even though his or her mother has been dead for many decades.

Of course, there is one major difference between the experience of a child and that of the older person or person with dementia, which is that the one is gradually learning and becoming more independent while the other is experiencing the opposite – gradually losing skills, capacities, knowledge.

There is a danger in taking this view, which is that dementia can be seen as a linear deterioration culminating in death. But dementia is not always like this, with the loss of language, for example, being interrupted by more lucid communication at times. Also, different forms of dementia can affect the language function in different ways.

This objection to seeing people with dementia as 'like children' is important because of the risk that if we treat someone like a child he or she will tend to behave like one. The belief that people with dementia are childlike can also reinforce a care approach that is authoritarian or rigid and that focuses on the loss of ability. This kind of care can infantilize and disempower the person with dementia.

Despite these risks, I think it can be helpful to explore this idea of the person with dementia becoming more childlike. In psychological terms, the unresolved emotional difficulties we experience in infancy and childhood can return in our adult lives. The person with dementia, like the young child, may have limited ability to make sense of or communicate his or her experience.

If it is true that the unresolved issues of infancy and childhood can return in dementia or older age, this allows us to view some of the unusual behaviour in a different way. The decay of cognitive abilities means the security of the person with dementia can feel threatened. This throws light on the common experience among those with dementia of fearing separation and abandonment. And just as a child can find it very difficult to have a succession of different carers or to move from familiar surroundings to unfamiliar ones, so the person with dementia can find it destabilizing to have a lack of consistency in his or her care and to be moved to a new, unfamiliar environment.

Child psychotherapist Margot Waddell, in her chapter in the book *Looking Into Later Life*, suggests that imagining how a child might feel in certain situations can help you if you are with the person with dementia.

For example, if the person with dementia becomes agitated or distressed when a loved one leaves the room, this can resemble the distress a young child might feel if his or her mother suddenly leaves – it represents a sudden loss of security. The message taken on by the person with dementia might be that he or she has been abandoned, that the loved one is never returning, that the person with dementia will henceforth have to survive alone.

What may be needed in this kind of situation, says Waddell, is a simple communication, like that which a mother would give her child, 'I'm just going to do X; I'll be back in a minute.'

17

Finding meaning in the experience

> Dementia does not teach you about the person with dementia, it teaches you about yourself.
>
> (John Suchet, *My Bonnie: How dementia stole the love of my life*)

It may seem strange to have a chapter exploring what, if any, are the positive sides of looking after a loved one with dementia. After all, dementia is a cruel, relentless illness that gradually destroys a person's brain and takes away his or her memories, physical capacities and identity.

I'm aware of the risk that, in reading these words, you may be thinking, 'What does he know? He hasn't been in my shoes, being treated aggressively by my husband and being accused of all kinds of things. And not being able to go out and have any independence because I have to look after him while he slowly gets worse and worse. Where's the "positive" in that?'

At the risk of being glib, and not wanting to minimize in any way the pain and stress that accompany looking after someone with dementia, my belief is that even the worst experiences can contain positive aspects, can contain meaning, even if these aspects are not clear at the time but only in retrospect.

I appreciate that this may be easier to recognize if the person with dementia you are close to does not show the aggressive, suspicious, cantankerous, even violent behaviour that some do. But even in these cases I think there is the possibility of something positive, or at least of making meaning out of the experience.

The degree to which we can make meaning out of this very difficult experience can be an important part of experiencing something positive. Again, when you are in the middle of the experience this may not be possible, but looking back you may find meaning in what you went through.

I want to stress that I am not talking here about 'focusing on the positive', trying to keep cheerful when everything feels as if it's falling apart, or counting your blessings even though you want to scream. The problem with that approach is that it can be superficial. While there is a clear role for appreciating what we do have and keeping sight of the positive, this approach can sometimes become a form of denial. The truth is that being close to someone who is gradually losing his or her mind is a very painful experience, particularly if that person is your parent, spouse, grandparent or other loved one.

No, what I am talking about here is something deeper, something that can be harder to put into words but is nevertheless real.

Finding meaning

Any major loss can activate the existential quest for meaning. It is in the most testing times of life that we can be forced to look at what the meaning of it all may be. This may be triggered by a death or a major change in our circumstances – something that stops us from carrying on our life as before.

In a way, it is not so important what meaning, if any, you ultimately find in the experience, but more the particular process you go through in getting to that place. The experience of caring for someone with dementia may lead you to ask questions about what really matters in life, such as:

- Who is the real me and what is the nature of identity and self?
- What really matters in life?
- What are my basic values and beliefs about the world?
- What do I want?

What we find out about ourselves

As the quote from John Suchet suggests, caring for or being close to a loved one with dementia teaches us an awful lot about ourselves. This is because it can be so challenging that it takes us to the edge of ourselves – showing us different parts of ourselves that we may not have been aware of, both in 'positive' and 'negative' ways.

By positive I am thinking of how we may discover reserves of patience or empathy or determination that we did not know we possessed.

On the other side, it can also make us aware of some less comfortable aspects of our character, such as our anger. While this does not sound 'positive', in the sense that it shows us that there is much more to us than we are consciously aware of, it can help us be more understanding to others who get caught up in similar emotions.

Love

One of the things we may find out about ourselves is how much love we have for the person with dementia. I don't mean love in the dewy-eyed Valentine's card sense, but the kind of love that involves commitment and courage. We may sometimes – even often –feel that we don't particularly like the person with dementia but we nevertheless have chosen to care for him or her and to do our best.

Looking after, or helping, the person with dementia gives us the opportunity to put into practice our love for that person. There are many definitions of love, but it seems to me that being willing to take care of someone with dementia, and make the inevitable sacrifices that brings, is part of love. We do it for a whole host of reasons and there may well be complex issues of duty or obligation and what we feel is expected of us. Nevertheless, at the heart of the experience is love for the other person, even though you may not always feel loved back.

This is, in many ways, a behaviour that goes against the emphasis on personal fulfilment and independence in our society. The idea of dutiful self-sacrifice for those we love seems rather old fashioned. Yet it is a very important idea.

Paula
Mum is now at the stage where she's not trusting me and that's painful. If she was an old lady who I had no connection with that wouldn't be too bad, but she's my mum. There have been a lot of downsides to looking after her, a lot of sacrifices, but I'm glad I did it. It's made me less selfish.

A deeper connection with the loved one may be possible

Dementia can allow a more simple, deeper connection with the loved one than we have become used to in the relationship. This may be particularly true in cases where there has been a difficult relationship in the past.

Nicola talks about her mother, a formerly busy and high-achieving woman who is now in the later stages of dementia, and with whom she did not share much physical affection in the past.

> Now I sit with her, taking her hand in mine, which I wouldn't have done before. When she was in the middle stage of dementia I would read her poetry – Tennyson, Wordsworth, Shakespeare – though I tried to avoid the topic of death in the poems I chose. I found that it was not so much what I said, but the way I said it that seemed to connect with her. I'd look into her eyes as I read and our relationship was intimate in a way that it wasn't before, but for a sad reason.

Many carers report that, alongside the frustrations and stresses, they also feel able to connect with the loved one in a simpler, deeper way. When it was a parent–child or husband–wife relationship, there were always complicated issues in the background and a sometimes difficult shared history.

It can bring families together

Although dementia can bring to the surface family tensions that may be covered over, it can sometimes have the opposite effect and enable families to become closer, even if only temporarily.

Claire
I've always had a difficult relationship with my brother, who was the favourite child of my mother's, and I ended up becoming her main carer when she got dementia. He was living abroad, but when he came over to help me clear out Mum's house and sort through her stuff we did become closer in that process, although it hasn't lasted as he's back abroad now.

It can lead to new interests or passions

The experience of looking after someone with dementia is often such an intense and emotionally challenging one that it can stimulate the carer to find new, creative ways of channelling his or her experiences.

This may include writing, such as a blog or poetry, or it could be painting or some other creative form of expression. Another way the experience can be channelled is through campaigning, such as for better dementia services.

Roberta, who has cared for her mother, has developed her photography hobby alongside a new interest in campaigning:

I had a terrible time early on, when Mum got dementia, because she had carers at her home and I was very busy with a teaching career, but there was no consistency in the agency carers – Mum had 35 different carers in six months – so I ended up living with Mum and becoming her carer.

While this meant a major sacrifice for me, it did mean that we ended up spending a lot of time together and it showed me how important our relationship was. If it hadn't been for the dementia I don't think we would have seen a huge amount of each other.

I'd always been interested in photography but when I found out that a friend of mine took photos of his father, who had dementia, I decided to do something similar with Mum and I also got involved with an organization campaigning for better social care. When I told them about my photography they supported me in putting on an exhibition and applying to the Arts Council for funding, so I recently had my first photographic exhibition.

Here are some of the ways you may find positives, or meaning, in the experience.

- You appreciate the fragility of life and therefore are able to live your own life to the full (when you are no longer in the caring role, of course).
- It puts into perspective the individualistic, youth-oriented and materialistic values common in many parts of society. It shows that there is another way to relate to each other that involves love, commitment and doing your best in very difficult circumstances.
- It enables you to learn new skills that you never needed before. Many men whose partners develop dementia may need to learn 'feminine' skills of cooking, housework, caring, while women may have to take more responsibility for traditionally 'masculine' roles such as the car, house maintenance, finances. Being allowed to take on these new roles, which otherwise would have remained rigidly associated with the man or woman, can bring new satisfactions.
- It can awaken a religious faith or, at the other extreme, convince you there is no God. In both ways this is part of the quest for meaning and making sense of the world in spiritual terms.

Staying in the present moment

Our true home is in the present moment. To live in the present moment is a miracle.

> (Thich Nhat Hanh, Zen Buddhist monk,
> author, teacher and peace activist)

One of the things learned by many people looking after someone with dementia is to try and stay in the present moment, because this is where people with dementia spend much of their time as memory falls away. Many of us are almost always busy. The challenges of being with a person with dementia can make you slow down and stay more in the present.

Spending time with a person with dementia, in which every day can seem like a new experience, can help us see that joy and laughter – as well as pain and anger – can all be experienced in the present moment without the usual reference points of the past and future which often dominate our thinking.

This is connected to the practice of mindfulness, which is about noticing what is happening in your present-moment experience, without judging it and without trying to change it.

If we can allow ourselves to enjoy the connection in the moment, without worrying so much about the future or past, there can be a space for something new. The person with dementia may quickly forget the connection, but in the moment it will be appreciated.

Appendix
Sources of support

Where to seek help

If you cannot take care of yourself you cannot take care of someone else, so it's crucial to find the support you need.

Not everyone wants support, of course. Many people prefer to get through it by themselves and hate the idea of talking to a professional, or even to friends or family, about what they see as private matters.

Lesley

I do find it distressing when my husband doesn't recognize our grandson any more, or that I can't leave him for more than an hour and a half without him coming to find me. But you just have to get on with life. I know there's support out there but I don't want to use it at the moment, I don't like to dwell on negative things.

But I would urge anyone who is struggling to find someone to talk to. That could be in person, on the phone or through an online support group. The phrase 'a problem shared is a problem halved' may be a cliché, but it does contain some truth.

Many carers may not want counselling but they do want to be able to tell their story without feeling judged or criticized. In these situations you will probably want to feel confident that you can talk without worrying that you are being 'too emotional' for the other person and having to take care of his or her feelings rather than stay in touch with your own.

Family and friends

Seeking support from other members of your family is an obvious place to start, although not always possible if you do not have other, supportive family members.

But for those that do, this is a crucial resource in providing support and helping you see your situation in a different light.

Fiona

My partner is very supportive and she is the one who tells me that I am taking on too much and I need to ask other relatives for help. Because I'm so immersed in the situation I can try to push myself too hard so it's very helpful to have another perspective from someone close to me.

Good friends, especially friends who have been through a similar experience, are also extremely valuable.

Anne

I sometimes get angry with Mum and then feel very guilty. What really helps is talking to a couple of close friends who have been through a similar process with relatives of their own. We share stories about how hard it is and that really helps me.

Roberta, whose mother has dementia, says:

I find it hard to ask for help, I've always been independent, but I'd advise anyone finding themselves in my situation to get support – from friends, family or agencies even if it means asking persistently. When I moved in at my mum's place I brought my own stuff, so then we had my stuff, Mum's and Dad's from when he was alive. I kept meaning to sort it all out but never had the time, so a friend suggested I invite her and some other friends over to help and that was fantastic.

Psychological family

The idea of our psychological family refers to those people who we can draw support from, who we can talk to and who we feel will listen without judgement. They may be members of our family but may also include friends, professionals, staff at a day centre, faith leaders or members of a support group. Other carers who you have developed a friendship with on internet forums may also be part of your psychological family.

If we don't feel we have a lot of support from our immediate family, thinking about who may be in our psychological family can help us identify sources of support.

Counselling and therapy

This may be needed if you find yourself really at a low ebb or, indeed, even if you feel you need to talk to someone to help make sense of a very difficult situation.

The main drawback to counselling and therapy is that if you are paying privately it is expensive and therefore not easily accessible for many people. But if you can afford it, or are willing to make sacrifices in other areas, it can be very helpful.

Claire, a middle-aged women whose mother had dementia, found herself as the main carer and having to sacrifice the development of her business. Her brother lived abroad.

> I felt I needed to talk to someone because I was carrying a heavy burden and feeling a lot of guilt that I wasn't doing enough. I was finding it really hard. I didn't want to confide in friends because I felt I'd be burdening them, or join a support group. I wanted to keep it private. I saw a therapist and that helped me lessen the burden and gave me somewhere to bring difficult feelings.

As well as private counselling, you may be able to access free or low-cost counselling from other sources. These include via your GP, from a local carers' organization or community counselling organization. Free or low-cost counselling will usually be limited to a certain number of sessions, such as six or ten. It is worth knowing that with community or carers' groups services you may be seeing a trainee or a counsellor with less experience.

Support groups and other meeting places

There are plenty of support groups out there, run by charities such as the Alzheimer's Society, Carers UK or local organizations. There are also other places where people with dementia and carers can socialize, such as dementia cafes.

Groups are an opportunity to hear the experiences of others who are in your position or have been there. You can also pick up practical tips on how to handle different situations or information about other services you may be entitled to.

Ruth
The carers group I'm in really helps because it makes me realize I'm not alone. It can be so easy to feel isolated and on your own in this situation.

Groups are also a good way of meeting others in a similar position to you.

Philippa
The local memory clinic ran a course of eight weekly sessions for carers and that was valuable. I also met a couple of people who I've stayed in touch with and it's great to be able to share experiences with them and have a bit of a laugh even if it's black humour.

Religion and spirituality

For some people the experience of looking after someone with dementia can push them away from an earlier religious belief, but for others it can awaken a religious, or spiritual, interest. That can take many forms, from traditional churches or religions to other forms of spirituality, such as meditation.

Making meaning out of the experience of caring is a continuing process, not something that is achieved and then complete. Being part of a religious or spiritual community can provide support in dealing with the questions and uncertainties that can arise from the experience.

The importance of respite

Having a break from looking after the person with dementia is hugely important, but can also be difficult because of financial and practical issues as well as the guilt that some carers feel about having other people look after the loved one.

Philippa
I've had two lots of two weeks of respite paid for by the local authority, where Mum went into a temporary home. She didn't get on that well in the first break, refusing to leave her room for most of the time. But it was great for me – I loved not having to worry about all the usual things and being able to visit friends I hadn't seen for ages because many of them live in other parts of the country. It felt like a huge weight lifted off me in that time.

Anti-depressants

Anti-depressants may be helpful for people who are really struggling. It is up to you as an individual to decide whether this is
something that you feel could help you, and where depression has
been long-running and seems intractable there may be a role for
such medication. As well as commercially produced pharmaceuti-
cals there are also herbal anti-depressants such as St John's Wort.

Useful addresses

Organizations for people with dementia

Admiral Nursing DIRECT
Helpline: 0845 257 9406 (9.15 a.m. to 4.45 p.m., Monday to Friday)
Email: direct@dementiauk.org
Website: www.dementiauk.org/information-support/admiral-nursing-direct

A national helpline and email service provided by **Dementia UK**. Experienced Admiral nurses offer practical advice and emotional support to people with dementia, those worried about memory loss, and their families and professional carers.

Alzheimer Scotland: Action on Dementia
22 Drumsheugh Gardens
Edinburgh EH3 7RN
Tel.: 0131 243 1453
Freephone helpline: 0808 808 3000 (24 hours)
Website: www.alzscot.org

Provides services, information and support for people with dementia and their families in Scotland.

Alzheimer's Disease International
64 Great Suffolk Street
London SE1 0BL
Tel.: 020 7981 0880
Website: www.alz.co.uk

ADI is the international federation of Alzheimer's associations around the world. It works by empowering local Alzheimer associations to promote and offer care and support for people with dementia and their carers, while working globally to focus attention on dementia.

Alzheimer's Society
Central office:
Devon House
58 St Katharine's Way
London E1W 1LB
National dementia helpline: 0300 222 11 22
Website: www.alzheimers.org.uk

Provides information and support for people with dementia and their families. There is a helpline, an online advice service and an online forum called 'Talking Point' for carers and family members.

AT Dementia
Trent Dementia Services Development Centre
Institute of Mental Health
University of Nottingham Innovation Park
Jubilee Campus
Triumph Road
Nottingham NG7 2TU
Tel.: 0115 748 4220
Website: www.atdementia.org.uk

Provides information on helpful ('assistive') technology for people with dementia.

Dementia UK
Second Floor
Resource for London
356 Holloway Road
London N7 6PA
Tel.: 020 7874 7200
Website: www.dementiauk.org

Dedicated to improving the quality of life for people with dementia. Dementia UK also provides Admiral nurses, who help families and carers of people with dementia, and **Admiral Nursing DIRECT**.

Frontotemporal Dementia Support Group (formerly Pick's Disease Support Group)
Website: www.ftdsg.org

NICE Guidance
Website: www.nice.org.uk/guidance/CG42

This document from the National Institute for Health and Care Excellence describes the treatment and support people with dementia can expect from the National Health Service and social services.

Organizations for carers

Care Quality Commission
CQC National Customer Service Centre
Citygate
Gallowgate
Newcastle-upon-Tyne NE1 4PA
Tel.: 03000 616161 (8.30 a.m. to 5.30 p.m., Monday to Friday)
Website: www.cqc.org.uk

Offers advice on choosing social care.

Carers Trust
32–6 Loman Street
London SE1 0EH
Te.l: 0844 800 4361
Website: www.carers.org

Enables carers to find local carers' centres or Crossroads (respite) care schemes.

Carers UK
20 Great Dover Street
London SE1 4LX
Tel.: 020 7378 4999
Helpline: 0808 808 7777
Website: www.carersuk.org

A campaigning group, national membership charity and support network for carers.

Crossroads Caring for Carers (Northern Ireland)
7 Regent Street
Newtownards BT23 4AB
Tel.: 028 9181 4455
Website: www.crossroadscare.co.uk

Provides respite care in the home to allow carers to take a break.

Crossroads Caring Scotland
Head office:
24 George Square
Glasgow G2 1EG
Tel.: 0141 226 3793
Website: www.crossroads-scotland.co.uk

Care and care homes

Barchester Healthcare Ltd
Head office:
Suite 201, Second Floor
Design Centre East
Chelsea Harbour
London SW10 0XF
Tel.: 0845 410 2828
Website: www.barchester.com

Offers a variety of types of care, including respite care and residential care.

Relatives' and Residents' Association
1 The Ivories
6–8 Northampton Street
London N1 2HY
Tel.: 020 7359 8148
Helpline: 020 7359 8136 (9.30 a.m. to 4.30 p.m., Monday to Friday)
Website: www.relres.org

Provides support with and information about going into residential care.

Sue Ryder Care
First Floor
16 Upper Woburn Place
London WC1H 0AF
Tel.: 0845 050 1953
Website: www.suerydercare.org

Provides residential care and support to older people with a range of life-changing conditions, including dementia.

Sunrise Senior Living
Sunrise House
Post Office Lane
Beaconsfield
Buckinghamshire HP9 1FN
Tel.: 0808 231 8554
Website: www.sunrise-care.co.uk

A care provider that has 27 residential communities in the UK, as well as others in the USA and Canada.

Holiday provision for people with disabilities

Enable holidays
Arion Business Centre
Harriett House
118 High Street
Erdington
Birmingham B23 6BG
Tel.: 0871 222 4939
Website: www.enableholidays.com

Offers information about holidays in Europe and the USA for people with special needs.

Revitalise
Head office:
212 Business Design Centre
52 Upper Street
London N1 0QH
Tel.: 0303 303 0145
Website: www.revitalise.org.uk

Provides holiday centres for people with disabilities, including dementia.

Other useful organizations

Age UK
Tavis House
1–6 Tavistock Square
London WC1H 9NA
Advice line: 0800 169 6565
Website: ageuk.org.uk

Provides information on all aspects of life for older people. The charity also provides information on and support for those affected by dementia, including an advice line on getting help from social services and a downloadable guide on caring for someone with dementia.

Citizens Advice
Tel.: 020 7833 2181 (administration only)
Website: www.citizensadvice.org.uk

Disabled Living Foundation
Ground Floor
Landmark House
Hammersmith Bridge Road
London W6 9EJ
Tel.: 020 7289 6111 (9 a.m. to 5 p.m., Monday to Friday)
Helpline: 0300 999 0004 (10 a.m. to 4 p.m., Monday to Friday)
Website: www.dlf.org.uk

Offers advice about helpful equipment for those with special needs.

Elizabeth Finn Care/Turn2us
Head office:
Hythe House
200 Shepherds Bush Road
London W6 7NL
Tel.: 020 8834 9200
Website: www.elizabethfinncare.org.uk

Provides grants for families in need.

Mental Health Foundation
Head office:
Colechurch House
1 London Bridge Walk
London SE1 2SX
Tel.: 020 7803 1100 (general enquiries); 020 7803 1101 (for publications)
Website: www.mentalhealth.org.uk

The Natural Death Centre
In The Hill House
Watley Lane
Twyford
Winchester SO21 1QX
Helpline: 01962 712690
Website: www.naturaldeath.org.uk

Provides information on advance directives or living wills.

Office of the Public Guardian
PO Box 16185
Birmingham B2 2WH
Tel.: 0300 456 0300 (9 a.m. to 5 p.m., Monday, Tuesday, Thursday, Friday;
10 a.m. to 5 p.m., Wednesday)
Website: www.publicguardian.gov.uk

Offers information about powers of attorney and the Court of Protection.

Relate
Tel.: 0300 100 1234
Website: www.relate.org.uk

Helps with all relationship problems.

Royal College of Psychiatrists
21 Prescot Street
London
E1 8BB
Tel.: 020 7235 2351; 020 7977 6655
Website: www.rcpsych.ac.uk

Produces leaflets on mental-health issues, including dementia.

Samaritans
Tel.: 08457 909090
Website: www.samaritans.org

A telephone support and listening service for those finding it difficult to cope.

References

Alzheimer's Disease International, *World Alzheimer Report 2012: Overcoming the stigma of dementia*. London: Alzheimer's Disease International, 2012.

Alzheimer's Australia, *Exploring Dementia and Stigma Beliefs: A pilot study of Australian adults aged 40 to 65 years*. Wollongong, NSW: University of Wollongong, 2012.

Balfour, Andrew, 'Facts, phenomenology, and psychoanalytic contributions to dementia care' in Rachael Davenhill (ed.) *Looking into Later Life: A psychoanalytic approach to depression and dementia in old age*. London: Karnac, 2007.

Bamford, Sally-Marie, *Women and Dementia – Not Forgotten*. London: ILC, 2011.

Bayley, John, *Iris: A memoir of Iris Murdoch*. London: Abacus, 1999.

Bouman, Walter Pierre, 'Sexuality and dementia', *Geriatric Medicine*. May 2007: 35–41.

Bowlby, John, *Attachment and Loss*, 3 volumes. London: Pimlico (Random House), 1997–8.

Capacchione, Lucia, *Recovery of Your Inner Child: The highly acclaimed method for liberating your inner self*. London: Simon and Schuster, 1991.

Carers UK, *Prepared to Care? Exploring the impact of caring on people's lives*. London: Carers UK, 2013.

Carling, Chris, *But Then Something Happened: A story of everyday dementia*. Cambridge: Golden Books, 2012.

Carroll, Claudia, 'Why do men expect their sisters to do all the caring?' *Daily Mail*, 17 January 2014.

Coon, David, Gallagher-Thompson, Dolores, and Thompson, Larry, *Innovative Interventions to Reduce Dementia Caregiver Stress: A clinical guide*. New York: Springer, 2003.

Daily Telegraph, 'Psychiatrists and nurses admit lying to dementia patients', 4 September 2013.

Davenhill, Rachael (ed.) *Looking into Later Life: A psychoanalytic approach to depression and dementia in old age*. London: Karnac, 2007.

Gillies, Andrea, *Keeper: A book about memory, identity, isolation, Wordsworth and cake*. London: Short Books, 2010.

Greenspan, Miriam, *Healing Through the Dark Emotions: The wisdom of grief, fear and despair*. Boston, Massachusetts: Shambhala Publications, 2004.

Harris Interactive, *What America Thinks: Metlife Foundation Alzheimer's Survey*, February 2011, available at: <www.metlife.com/assets/cao/foundation/alzheimers-2011.pdf>.

ILC-UK, *The Last Taboo: A guide to dementia, sexuality, intimacy and sexual behaviour in care homes*. London: ILC, 2011.

James, Oliver, *Contented Dementia: 24-hour wraparound care for lifelong well-being*. London: Vermilion, 2009.

Karpman, Stephen, 'Fairy tales and script drama analysis', *Transactional Analysis Bulletin* 7.26 (1968): 39–43.

Kitwood, Tom, *Dementia Reconsidered: The person comes first*. Oxford: Oxford University Press, 1997.

Lorenz, Konrad, *The Year of the Greylag Goose*. Orlando, Florida: Harcourt Brace Jovanovich, 1979.

Oyebode, Jan, 'Assessment of carers' psychological needs', *Advances in Psychiatric Treatment* 9 (2003): 45–53.

Phillips, Fiona, *Before I Forget: A daughter's story*. London: Cornerstone, 2010.

Real, Terrence, *How Can I Get Through to You? Closing the intimacy gap between men and women*. London: Simon & Schuster, 2003.

Richo, David, *How to Be an Adult: A handbook on psychological and spiritual integration*. Mahwah, New Jersey: Paulist Press, 1991.

Slevin, Martin, *The Little Girl in the Radiator*. Cheltenham: Monday Books, 2012.

Stone, Hal and Sidra, *Embracing Our Selves: The voice dialogue manual*. San Francisco: New World Library, 1998.

Suchet, John, *My Bonnie: How dementia stole the love of my life*. London: Harper, 2010.

Talbot, Marianne, *Keeping Mum: Caring for someone with dementia*. London: Hay House UK, 2011.

Taylor, Richard, *Alzheimer's From the Inside Out*. Baltimore, Maryland: Health Professions Press, 2007.

Waddell, Margot, 'Only connect – the links between early and later life' in Rachael Davenhill (ed.) *Looking into Later Life: A psychoanalytic approach to depression and dementia in old age*. London: Karnac, 2007.

Williams, Mark, Teasdale, John, Segal, Zindel, and Kabat-Zinn, Jon, *The Mindful Way Through Depression: Freeing yourself from chronic unhappiness*. New York: Guilford Press, 2007.

Witchel, Alex, 'How dementia changes families', *AARP: The Magazine*, available at: <http://www.aarp.org/home-family/caregiving/info-03-2013/symptoms-dementia-alzheimers-memory-loss.html>.

Wood, Heather, 'Caring for a relative with dementia: who is the sufferer?' in Rachael Davenhill (ed.) *Looking into Later Life: A psychoanalytic approach to depression and dementia in old age*. London: Karnac, 2007.

Worden, William, *Grief Counselling and Grief Therapy: A handbook for the mental health practitioner*. London: Routledge, 2009 (fourth edition).

Wright, L. K., 'The impact of Alzheimer's disease on the marital relationship', *The Gerontologist* 31.2 (1991): 224–37.

Wright, L. K. 'Alzheimer's Disease afflicted spouses who remain at home', *Social Sciences and Medicine* 38.8 (1994): 1037–46.

Index